Ben Stacy Jerrik (Ed.)

Telecare

Ben Stacy Jerrik (Ed.)

Telecare

Dementia, Safety Confirmation, Telemedicine, Telehealth

Part Press

Imprint

Publisher:
Part Press is a trademark of
International Book Market Service Ltd., 17 Rue Meldrum, Beau Bassin, 1713-01 Mauritius
Email: info@bookmarketservice.com
Website: www.bookmarketservice.com

Published in 2011

Printed in: U.S.A., U.K., Germany. This book was not produced in Mauritius.

ISBN: 978-613-8-94615-1

Contents

Articles

References

Telecare

Telecare is a term given to offering remote care of old and physically less able people, providing the care and reassurance needed to allow them to remain living in their own homes. The use of sensors may be part of a package which can provide support for people with illnesses such as dementia, or people at risk of falling. In 2005 the UK's Department of Health published *Building Telecare in England* to coincide with the announcement of a grant to help encourage its take up by local councils with social care responsibilities.[1]

Most telecare mitigates harm by reacting to untoward events and raising a help response quickly. Some telecare, such as safety confirmation and lifestyle monitoring have a preventive function in that a deterioration in the telecare user's wellbeing can be spotted at an early stage.

Telecare is specifically different from telemedicine and telehealth. Telecare refers to the idea of enabling people to remain independent in their own homes by providing person-centred technologies to support the individual or their carers.

In its simplest form, it can refer to a fixed or mobile telephone with a connection to a monitoring centre through which the user can raise an alarm. Technologically more advanced systems use sensors, whereby a range of potential risks can be monitored. These may include falls, as well as environmental changes in the home such as floods, fire and gas leaks. Carers of people with dementia my be alerted if the person leaves the house or other defined area. When a sensor is activated it sends a radio signal to a central unit in the user's home, which then automatically calls a 24-hour monitoring centre where trained operators can take appropriate action, whether it be contacting a local key holder, doctor or the emergency services.

Telecare also comprises standalone telecare which does not send signals to a response centre but supports carers through providing local (in-house) alerts in a person's home to let the carer know when a person requires attention.

The meaning and usage of the term 'telecare' has not yet settled into consistent use. In the UK it is grounded in the social care framework and focuses on the meaning described above. In other countries 'telecare' may be applied to the practice of healthcare at a distance.

Technological advances result in the possibility of promoting independence and for providing care from the social initiative sector, which now contemplates eCare, and navigation/positioning systems, such as GPS for people with dementia or other cognitive impairments.

It is important to note that 'telecare' is not just a warning system if someone strays from home but is also preventative measure whereby people are brought back and kept in the community through regular communication.[2]

There are now a large range of telecare services available with some of the most well known being the pendant alarm[3] , pill dispenser[4] , telephone prompt service [5] , the movement monitoring[6] and more. All play a role in maintaining people's independence and allowing people to stay in their own homes.

See also

- Assistive technology
- Wandering (dementia)

References

[1] Building Telecare in England (http://www.dh.gov.uk/en/Publicationsandstatistics/Publications/PublicationsPolicyAndGuidance/DH_4115303)
[2] Independent Living Telecare (http://www.independentliving.co.uk/telecare.html)
[3] Tunstall - Pendant Alarm (http://www.tunstall.co.uk)
[4] Pivotell - Pill Dispenser (http://www.pivotell.co.uk)
[5] Telecare Technology - Telephone Prompt Service (http://www.telecaretechnology.com)
[6] Just Checking - Movement Monitoring (http://www.justchecking.co.uk)

External links

- International Society for Telemedicine & eHealth (http://www.isft.net/)

Sensor

A **sensor** (also called **detector**) is a device that measures a physical quantity and converts it into a signal which can be read by an observer or by an instrument. For example, a mercury-in-glass thermometer converts the measured temperature into expansion and contraction of a liquid which can be read on a calibrated glass tube. A thermocouple converts temperature to an output voltage which can be read by a voltmeter. For accuracy, most sensors are calibrated against known standards.

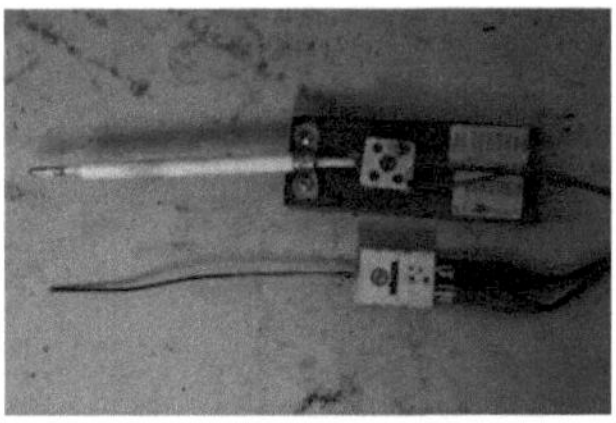

Thermocouple sensor for high temperature measurement

Use

Sensors are used in everyday objects such as touch-sensitive elevator buttons (tactile sensor) and lamps which dim or brighten by touching the base. There are also innumerable applications for sensors of which most people are never aware. Applications include cars, machines, aerospace, medicine, manufacturing and robotics.

A sensor is a device which receives and responds to a signal. A sensor's sensitivity indicates how much the sensor's output changes when the measured quantity changes. For instance, if the mercury in a thermometer moves 1 cm when the temperature changes by 1 °C, the sensitivity is 1 cm/°C (it is basically the slope Dy/Dx assuming a linear characteristic). Sensors that measure very small changes must have very high sensitivities. Sensors also have an impact on what they measure; for instance, a room temperature thermometer inserted into a hot cup of liquid cools the liquid while the liquid heats the thermometer. Sensors need to be designed to have a small effect on what is measured; making the sensor smaller often improves this and may introduce other advantages. Technological progress allows more and more sensors to be manufactured on a microscopic scale as microsensors using MEMS technology. In most cases, a microsensor reaches a significantly higher speed and sensitivity compared with macroscopic approaches.

Classification of measurement errors

A good sensor obeys the following rules:

- Is sensitive to the measured property only
- Is insensitive to any other property likely to be encountered in its application
- Does not influence the measured property

Ideal sensors are designed to be linear or linear to some simple mathematical function of the measurement, typically logarithmic. The output signal of such a sensor is linearly proportional to the value or simple function of the measured property. The sensitivity is then defined as the ratio between output signal and measured property. For example, if a sensor measures temperature and has a voltage output, the sensitivity is a constant with the unit [V/K]; this sensor is linear because the ratio is constant at all points of measurement.

Sensor deviations

If the sensor is not ideal, several types of deviations can be observed:

- The sensitivity may in practice differ from the value specified. This is called a sensitivity error, but the sensor is still linear.
- Since the range of the output signal is always limited, the output signal will eventually reach a minimum or maximum when the measured property exceeds the limits. The full scale range defines the maximum and minimum values of the measured property.
- If the output signal is not zero when the measured property is zero, the sensor has an offset or bias. This is defined as the output of the sensor at zero input.
- If the sensitivity is not constant over the range of the sensor, this is called non linearity. Usually this is defined by the amount the output differs from ideal behavior over the full range of the sensor, often noted as a percentage of the full range.
- If the deviation is caused by a rapid change of the measured property over time, there is a dynamic error. Often, this behavior is described with a bode plot showing sensitivity error and phase shift as function of the frequency of a periodic input signal.
- If the output signal slowly changes independent of the measured property, this is defined as drift (telecommunication).
- Long term drift usually indicates a slow degradation of sensor properties over a long period of time.
- Noise is a random deviation of the signal that varies in time.
- Hysteresis is an error caused by when the measured property reverses direction, but there is some finite lag in time for the sensor to respond, creating a different offset error in one direction than in the other.
- If the sensor has a digital output, the output is essentially an approximation of the measured property. The approximation error is also called digitization error.
- If the signal is monitored digitally, limitation of the sampling frequency also can cause a dynamic error, or if the variable or added noise noise changes periodically at a frequency near a multiple of the sampling rate may induce aliasing errors.
- The sensor may to some extent be sensitive to properties other than the property being measured. For example, most sensors are influenced by the temperature of their environment.

All these deviations can be classified as systematic errors or random errors. Systematic errors can sometimes be compensated for by means of some kind of calibration strategy. Noise is a random error that can be reduced by signal processing, such as filtering, usually at the expense of the dynamic behavior of the sensor.

Resolution

The resolution of a sensor is the smallest change it can detect in the quantity that it is measuring. Often in a digital display, the least significant digit will fluctuate, indicating that changes of that magnitude are only just resolved. The resolution is related to the precision with which the measurement is made. For example, a scanning tunneling probe (a fine tip near a surface collects an electron tunnelling current) can resolve atoms and molecules.

Sensors in Nature

Further information: Sense

All living organisms contain biological sensors with functions similar to those of the mechanical devices described. Most of these are specialized cells that are sensitive to:

- Light, motion, temperature, magnetic fields, gravity, humidity, moisture, vibration, pressure, electrical fields, sound, and other physical aspects of the external environment
- Physical aspects of the internal environment, such as stretch, motion of the organism, and position of appendages (proprioception)
- Environmental molecules, including toxins, nutrients, and pheromones
- Estimation of biomolecules interaction and some kinetics parameters
- Internal metabolic milieu, such as glucose level, oxygen level, or osmolality
- Internal signal molecules, such as hormones, neurotransmitters, and cytokines
- Differences between proteins of the organism itself and of the environment or alien creatures.

Biosensor

In biomedicine and biotechnology, sensors which detect analytes thanks to a biological component, such as cells, protein, nucleic acid or biomimetic polymers, are called biosensors. Whereas a non-biological sensor, even organic (=carbon chemistry), for biological analytes is referred to as sensor or nanosensor (such a microcantilevers). This terminology applies for both in vitro and in vivo applications. The encapsulation of the biological component in biosensors, presents with a slightly different problem that ordinary sensors, this can either be done by means of a semipermeable barrier, such as a dialysis membrane or a hydrogel, a 3D polymer matrix, which either physically constrains the sensing macromolecule or chemically (macromolecule is bound to the scaffold).[1]

See also

- Actuator
- Capacitive displacement sensor
- Data acquisition
- Data logger
- Detection theory
- Fully automatic time
- Lateral line
- Leaf sensor
- Limen
- Machine olfaction
- Nanoelectronics
- Nanosensor
- Printed electronics
- Receiver operating characteristic
- Transducer

- Wireless sensor network
- Sensor web

References

[1] Wolfbeis, O. S. (2000). "Fiber-optic chemical sensors and biosensors." Anal Chem 72(12): 81R-89R

External links

- Capacitive Position/Displacement Sensor Theory/Tutorial (http://www.capsensortheory.com)
- Capacitive Position/Displacement Overview (http://www.capsensors.com)
- Comparing Capacitive and Eddy-Current Sensors (http://www.lionprecision.com/tech-library/technotes/article-0011-cve.html)
- M. Kretschmar and S. Welsby (2005), Capacitive and Inductive Displacement Sensors, in Sensor Technology Handbook, J. Wilson editor, Newnes: Burlington, MA.
- C. A. Grimes, E. C. Dickey, and M. V. Pishko (2006), Encyclopedia of Sensors (10-Volume Set), American Scientific Publishers. ISBN 1-58883-056-X
- Sensors (http://www.mdpi.com/journal/sensors) - Open access journal of MDPI (http://www.mdpi.net)
- M. Pohanka, O. Pavlis, and P. Skladal. Rapid Characterization of Monoclonal Antibodies using the Piezoelectric Immunosensor (http://www.mdpi.org/sensors/papers/s7030341.pdf). *Sensors* 2007, **7**, 341-353
- SensEdu; how sensors work (http://www.sensedu.com/)
- Clifford K. Ho, Alex Robinson, David R. Miller and Mary J. Davis. Overview of Sensors and Needs for Environmental Monitoring (http://www.mdpi.net/sensors/papers/s5010004.pdf). *Sensors* 2005, **5**, 4-37
- Wireless hydrogen sensor (http://news.ufl.edu/2006/05/24/hydrogen-sensor/)
- Sensors and Actuators A: Physical (http://www.elsevier.com/wps/find/journaldescription.cws_home/504103/description#description) - Elsevier journal
- Sensors and Actuators B: Chemical (http://www.elsevier.com/wps/find/journaldescription.cws_home/504104/description#description) - Elsevier journal
- Automotive Electronic Sensors (http://www.cvel.clemson.edu/auto/sensors/auto-sensors.html)

Dementia

Dementia	
Classification and external resources	
ICD-10	F00 [1]-F07 [2]
ICD-9	290 [3]-294 [4]
DiseasesDB	29283 [5]
MedlinePlus	000739 [6]
MeSH	D003704 [7]

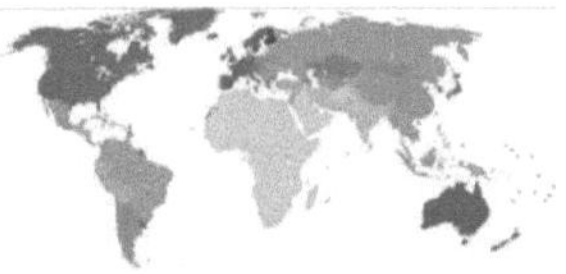

Disability-adjusted life year for Alzheimer and other dementias per 100,000 inhabitants in 2002. no data ≤ 50 50-70 70-90 90-110 110-130 130-150 150-170 170-190 190-210 210-230 230-250 ≥ 250

Dementia (taken from Latin, originally meaning "madness", from *de-* "without" + *ment*, the root of *mens* "mind") is a serious loss of cognitive ability in a previously unimpaired person, beyond what might be expected from normal aging. It may be static, the result of a unique global brain injury, or progressive, resulting in long-term decline due to damage or disease in the body. Although dementia is far more common in the geriatric population, it can occur before the age of 65, in which case it is termed "early onset dementia".[8]

Dementia is not a single disease, but rather a non-specific illness syndrome (i.e., set of signs and symptoms) in which affected areas of cognition may be memory, attention, language, and problem solving. It is normally required to be present for at least 6 months to be diagnosed;[9] cognitive dysfunction that has been seen only over shorter times, in particular less than weeks, must be termed delirium. In all types of general cognitive dysfunction, higher mental functions are affected first in the process.

Especially in the later stages of the condition, affected persons may be disoriented in time (not knowing what day of the week, day of the month, or even what year it is), in place (not knowing where they are), and in person (not knowing who they, or others around them, are). Dementia, though often treatable to some degree, is usually due to causes that are progressive and incurable.

Symptoms of dementia can be classified as either reversible or irreversible, depending upon the etiology of the disease. Less than 10% of cases of dementia are due to causes that may presently be reversed with treatment. Causes include many different specific disease processes, in the same way that symptoms of organ dysfunction such as shortness of breath, jaundice, or pain are attributable to many etiologies.

Without careful assessment of history, the short-term syndrome of delirium (often lasting days to weeks) can easily be confused with dementia, because they have all symptoms in common, save duration. Some mental illnesses, including depression and psychosis, may produce symptoms that must be differentiated from both delirium and dementia.[10]

There are many specific types (causes) of dementia, often showing slightly different symptoms. However, the symptom overlap is such that it is impossible to diagnose the type of dementia by symptomatology alone, and in only a few cases are symptoms enough to give a high probability of some specific cause. Diagnosis is therefore aided by nuclear medicine brain scanning techniques. Certainty cannot be attained except with brain biopsy during life, or at necropsy in death.

Some of the most common forms of dementia are: Alzheimer's disease, vascular dementia, frontotemporal dementia, semantic dementia and dementia with Lewy bodies. It is possible for a patient to exhibit two or more dementing processes at the same time, as none of the known types of dementia protects against the others.

History

Up to the end of the 19th century, dementia was a much broader clinical concept, which included mental illness and any type of psychosocial incapacity, including those which could be reversed.[11] Dementia at this time simply referred to anyone who had lost the ability to reason, and was applied equally to psychosis of mental illness, "organic" diseases like syphilis which could destroy the brain, and to the dementia associated with old age, which was held to be caused by "hardening of the arteries."

Dementia when seen in the elderly was called **senile dementia** or **senility** and viewed as a normal and somewhat inevitable aspect of growing old, rather than as being caused by any specific diseases. At the same time, in 1907, a specific organic dementing process of early onset, called Alzheimer's disease, had been described. This was associated with particular microscopic changes in the brain, but was seen as a rare disease of middle age.

Much like other diseases associated with aging, dementia was rare before the 20th century, although by no means unknown, due to the fact that people seldom lived long enough to experience it.

By the period of 1913-20, schizophrenia had been well-defined in a way similar to today, and also the term dementia praecox had been used to suggest the development of senile-type dementia at a younger age. Eventually the two terms fused, so that until 1952 physicians used the terms dementia praecox ("precocious dementia") and schizophrenia interchangeably. The term "precocious dementia" for a mental illness suggested that a type of mental illness like schizophrenia (including paranoia and decreased cognitive capacity) could be expected to arrive normally in all persons with greater age (see paraphrenia). At the same time, the beginning use of dementia to describe both what we know understand as schizophrenia and senile dementia, after about 1920, acted to give the word "dementia" a more limited role, as one of describing a type of permanent mental deterioration which was not expected to be reversible. This is the beginning of the more recognizable use of the term today.

In 1976, neurologist Robert Katzmann suggested a link between "senile dementia" and Alzheimer's disease.[12] Katzmann suggested that much of the senile dementia occurring (by definition) after the age of 65, was pathologically identical with Alzheimer's disease occurring before age 65 and therefore should not be treated differently. He noted that the fact the "senile dementia" was not considered a disease, but rather part of aging, and this fact was keeping millions of aged patients with what otherwise was identical with Alzheimer's disease, from being diagnosed as having a disease process, rather than simply considered as aging normally.[13] Katzmann thus suggested that Alzheimer's disease, if taken to occur over age 65, is actually common, not rare, and was the 4th or 5th leading cause of death, even though rarely being reported on death certificates in 1976.

This suggestion opened the view that dementia is never normal, and must always be the result of a particular disease process, and is not part of the normal healthy aging process, *per se*. The ensuing debate led for a time to the proposed disease diagnosis of "senile dementia of the Alzheimer's type" (SDAT) in persons over the age of 65, with "Alzheimer's disease" diagnosed in persons younger than 65 who had the same pathology. Eventually, however, it was agreed that the age limit was artificial, and that Alzheimer's disease was the appropriate term for persons with the particular brain pathology seen in this disease, regardless of the age of the sufferer. A helpful finding was that although the incidence of Alzheimer's disease increased with age (from 5-10% of 75-year-olds to as many as 40-50% of 90-year-olds), there was no age at which all persons developed it, so it was not an inevitable consequence of aging, no matter how great an age a person attained.

Also, after 1952, mental illnesses like schizophrenia were removed from the category of "organic brain syndromes," and thus (by definition) removed from possible causes of "dementing illnesses" (dementias). At the same, however, the traditional cause of senile dementia – "hardening of the arteries" – now returned as a set of dementias of vascular cause (small strokes). These were now termed "multi-infarct dementias" or vascular dementias.

In the 21st century, a number of other types of dementia have been differentiated from Alzheimer's disease and vascular dementias (these two being the most common types). This differentiation is on the basis of pathological examination of brain tissues, symptomatology, and by different patterns of brain metabolic activity in nuclear medical imaging tests such as SPECT and PET scans of the brain. The various forms of dementia have differing prognoses (expected outcome of illness), and also differing sets of epidemologic risk factors. The causal etiology of many of them, including Alzheimer's disease, remains unknown, although many theories exist such as accumulation of protein plaques as part of normal aging, inflammation, inadequate blood sugar, and traumatic brain injury.

Signs and symptoms

Comorbidities

Dementia is not merely a problem of memory. It reduces the ability to learn, reason, retain or recall past experience and there is also loss of patterns of thoughts, feelings and activities (Gelder *et al.* 2005). Additional mental and behavioral problems often affect people who have dementia, and may influence quality of life, caregivers, and the need for institutionalization. As dementia worsens individuals may neglect themselves and may become disinhibited and may become incontinent. (Gelder *et al.* 2005).

Depression affects 20–30% of people who have dementia, and about 20% have anxiety.[14] Psychosis (often delusions of persecution) and agitation/aggression also often accompany dementia. Each of these needs to be assessed and treated independent of the underlying dementia.[15]

Risk to self and others

The Canadian Medical Association Journal has reported that driving with dementia could lead to severe injury or even death to self and others. Doctors should advise appropriate testing on when to quit driving.[16]

In the United States, Florida's Baker Act allows law enforcement and the judiciary to force mental evaluation for those suspected of suffering from dementia or other mental incapacities.

In the United Kingdom, as with all mental disorders, where a sufferer could potentially be a danger to themselves or others, they can be detained under the Mental Health Act of 1983 for the purposes of assessment, care and treatment. This is a last resort, and usually avoided if the patient has family or friends who can ensure care.

The United Kingdom DVLA (Driving & Vehicle Licensing Agency) states that dementia sufferers who specifically suffer with poor short term memory, disorientation, lack of insight or judgment are almost certainly not fit to drive—and in these instances, the DVLA must be informed so said license can be revoked. They do however acknowledge low-severity cases and early sufferers, and those drivers may be permitted to drive pending medical reports.

Behaviour may be disorganized, restless or inappropriate. Some people become restless or wander about by day and sometimes at night. When people suffering from dementia are put in circumstances beyond their abilities, there may be a sudden change to tears or anger (a *"catastrophic reaction"*).[17]

Causes

Fixed cognitive impairment

Various types of brain injury, occurring as a single event, may cause irreversible but fixed cognitive impairment. Traumatic brain injury may cause generalized damage to the white matter of the brain (diffuse axonal injury), or more localized damage (as also may neurosurgery). A temporary reduction in the brain's supply of blood or oxygen may lead to hypoxic-ischemic injury. Strokes (ischemic stroke, or intracerebral, subarachnoid, subdural or extradural hemorrhage) or infections (meningitis and/or encephalitis) affecting the brain, prolonged epileptic seizures and acute hydrocephalus may also have long-term effects on cognition. Excessive alcohol use may cause alcohol dementia, Wernicke's encephalopathy and/or Korsakoff's psychosis, and certain other recreational drugs may cause substance-induced persisting dementia; once overuse ceases, the cognitive impairment is persistent but not progressive.

Slowly progressive dementia

Dementia which begins gradually and worsens progressively over several years is usually caused by neurodegenerative disease; that is, by conditions affecting only or primarily the neurons of the brain and causing gradual but irreversible loss of function of these cells. Less commonly, a non-degenerative condition may have secondary effects on brain cells, which may or may not be reversible if the condition is treated.

The causes of dementia depend on the age at which symptoms begin. In the elderly population (usually defined in this context as over 65 years of age), a large majority of cases of dementia are caused by Alzheimer's disease, vascular dementia or both. Dementia with Lewy bodies is another fairly common cause, which again may occur alongside either or both of the other causes.[18] [19] [20] Hypothyroidism sometimes causes slowly progressive cognitive impairment as the main symptom, and this may be fully reversible with treatment. Normal pressure hydrocephalus, though relatively rare, is important to recognize since treatment may prevent progression and improve other symptoms of the condition. However, significant cognitive improvement is unusual.

Dementia is much less common under 65 years of age. Alzheimer's disease is still the most frequent cause, but inherited forms of the disease account for a higher proportion of cases in this age group. Frontotemporal lobar degeneration and Huntington's disease account for most of the remaining cases.[21] Vascular dementia also occurs, but this in turn may be due to underlying conditions (including antiphospholipid syndrome, CADASIL, MELAS, homocystinuria, moyamoya and Binswanger's disease). People who receive frequent head trauma, such as boxers or football players, are at risk of chronic traumatic encephalopathy[22] (also called dementia pugilistica in boxers).

In young adults (up to 40 years of age) who were previously of normal intelligence, it is very rare to develop dementia without other features of neurological disease, or without features of disease elsewhere in the body. Most cases of progressive cognitive disturbance in this age group are caused by psychiatric illness, alcohol or other drugs, or metabolic disturbance. However, certain genetic disorders can cause true neurodegenerative dementia at this age. These include familial Alzheimer's disease, SCA17 (dominant inheritance); adrenoleukodystrophy (X-linked); Gaucher's disease type 3, metachromatic leukodystrophy, Niemann-Pick disease type C, pantothenate kinase-associated neurodegeneration, Tay-Sachs disease and Wilson's disease (all recessive). Wilson's disease is particularly important since cognition can improve with treatment.

At all ages, a substantial proportion of patients who complain of memory difficulty or other cognitive symptoms are suffering from depression rather than a neurodegenerative disease. Vitamin deficiencies and chronic infections may also occur at any age; they usually cause other symptoms before dementia occurs, but occasionally mimic degenerative dementia. These include deficiencies of vitamin B_{12}, folate or niacin, and infective causes including cryptococcal meningitis, HIV, Lyme disease, progressive multifocal leukoencephalopathy, subacute sclerosing panencephalitis, syphilis and Whipple's disease.

Rapidly progressive dementia

Creutzfeldt-Jakob disease typically causes a dementia which worsens over weeks to months, being caused by prions. The common causes of slowly progressive dementia also sometimes present with rapid progression: Alzheimer's disease, dementia with Lewy bodies, frontotemporal lobar degeneration (including corticobasal degeneration and progressive supranuclear palsy).

On the other hand, encephalopathy or delirium may develop relatively slowly and resemble dementia. Possible causes include brain infection (viral encephalitis, subacute sclerosing panencephalitis, Whipple's disease) or inflammation (limbic encephalitis, Hashimoto's encephalopathy, cerebral vasculitis); tumors such as lymphoma or glioma; drug toxicity (e.g. anticonvulsant drugs); metabolic causes such as liver failure or kidney failure; and chronic subdural hematoma.

Dementia as a feature of other conditions

There are many other medical and neurological conditions in which dementia only occurs late in the illness, or as a minor feature. For example, a proportion of patients with Parkinson's disease develop dementia, though widely varying figures are quoted for this proportion. When dementia occurs in Parkinson's disease, the underlying cause may be dementia with Lewy bodies or Alzheimer's disease, or both.[23] Cognitive impairment also occurs in the Parkinson-plus syndromes of progressive supranuclear palsy and corticobasal degeneration (and the same underlying pathology may cause the clinical syndromes of frontotemporal lobar degeneration). Chronic inflammatory conditions of the brain may affect cognition in the long term, including Behçet's disease, multiple sclerosis, sarcoidosis, Sjögren's syndrome and systemic lupus erythematosus. Although the acute porphyrias may cause episodes of confusion and psychiatric disturbance, dementia is a rare feature of these rare diseases.[24]

Aside from those mentioned above, inherited conditions which may cause dementia alongside other features include:[25]

- Alexander disease
- Canavan disease
- Cerebrotendinous xanthomatosis
- DRPLA
- Fragile X-associated tremor/ataxia syndrome
- Glutaric aciduria type 1
- Krabbe's disease
- Maple syrup urine disease
- Niemann Pick disease type C
- Kufs' disease
- Neuroacanthocytosis
- Organic acidemias
- Pelizaeus-Merzbacher disease
- Urea cycle disorders
- Sanfilippo syndrome type B
- Spinocerebellar ataxia type 2

Diagnosis

Proper differential diagnosis between the types of dementia (cortical and subcortical) will require, at the least, referral to a specialist, e.g., a geriatric internist, geriatric psychiatrist, neurologist, neuropsychologist or geropsychologist. Duration of symptoms must evident for at least six months for a diagnosis of dementia or organic brain syndrome to be made (ICD-10).

Cognitive testing

Sensitivity and specificity of common tests for dementia

Test	Sensitivity	Specificity	Reference
MMSE	71%-92%	56%-96%	[26]
3MS	83%-93.5%	85%-90%	[27]
AMTS	73%-100%	71%-100%	[27]

There exist some brief tests (5–15 minutes) that have reasonable reliability and can be used in the office or other setting to screen cognitive status. Examples of such tests include the abbreviated mental test score (AMTS), the mini mental state examination (MMSE), *Modified Mini-Mental State Examination* (3MS),[28] the *Cognitive Abilities Screening Instrument* (CASI),[29] and the clock drawing test.[30] Scores must be interpreted in the context of the person's educational and other background, and the particular circumstances; for example, a person highly depressed or in great pain will not be expected to do well on many tests of mental ability.

While many tests have been studied,[31] [32] [33] and some may emerge as better alternatives to the MMSE, presently the MMSE is the best studied and most commonly used.

Another approach to screening for dementia is to ask an informant (relative or other supporter) to fill out a questionnaire about the person's everyday cognitive functioning. Informant questionnaires provide complementary information to brief cognitive tests. Probably the best known questionnaire of this sort is the *Informant Questionnaire on Cognitive Decline in the Elderly (IQCODE)*.[34] On the other hand the *General Practitioner Assessment Of Cognition* combines both, a patient assessment and an informant interview. It was specifically designed for the use in the primary care setting and is also available as a web-based test.

Further evaluation includes retesting at another date, and administration of other tests of mental function.

Laboratory tests

Routine blood tests are also usually performed to rule out treatable causes. These tests include vitamin B_{12}, folic acid, thyroid-stimulating hormone (TSH), C-reactive protein, full blood count, electrolytes, calcium, renal function, and liver enzymes. Abnormalities may suggest vitamin deficiency, infection or other problems that commonly cause confusion or disorientation in the elderly. The problem is complicated by the fact that these cause confusion more often in persons who have early dementia, so that "reversal" of such problems may ultimately only be temporary.

Testing for alcohol and other known dementia-inducing drugs may be indicated.

Imaging

A CT scan or magnetic resonance imaging (MRI scan) is commonly performed, although these modalities do not have optimal sensitivity for the diffuse metabolic changes associated with dementia in a patient that shows no gross neurological problems (such as paralysis or weakness) on neurological exam. CT or MRI may suggest normal pressure hydrocephalus, a potentially reversible cause of dementia, and can yield information relevant to other types of dementia, such as infarction (stroke) that would point at a vascular type of dementia.

The functional neuroimaging modalities of SPECT and PET are more useful in assessing long-standing cognitive dysfunction, since they have shown similar ability to diagnose dementia as a clinical exam.[35] The ability of SPECT to differentiate the vascular cause from the Alzheimer's disease cause of dementias, appears to be superior to differentiation by clinical exam.[36]

Recent research has established the value of PET imaging using carbon-11 Pittsburgh Compound B as a radiotracer (PIB-PET) in predictive diagnosis of various kinds of dementia, in particular Alzheimer's disease. Studies from Australia have found PIB-PET to be 86% accurate in predicting which patients with mild cognitive impairment would develop Alzheimer's disease within two years. In another study, carried out using 66 patients seen at the University of Michigan, PET studies using either PIB or another radiotracer, carbon-11 dihydrotetrabenazine (DTBZ), led to more accurate diagnosis for more than one-fourth of patients with mild cognitive impairment or mild dementia.[37]

Prevention

A study done at the University of Bari in Italy, found that a group drinking alcoholic beverages moderately had a slower progression to dementia. In a group of 1,566 elderly Italians, 1,445 had no cognitive impairment and 121 had suffered mild cognitive impairment, the study found that that over the duration of 3.5 years the people with MCI who drank less than one alcoholic beverage a day progressed to dementia at a rate that was 85% slower then those who drank no alcoholic beverages. However, the authors of the study commented that since it was epidemiologic, the findings might only be a marker of lifestyle, showing that "moderate lifestyle" in general is associated with slower dementia-progression.[38] A study failed to show a conclusive link between high blood pressure and developing dementia. The study, published in the *Lancet Neurology* journal July 2008, found that blood pressure lowering medication did not reduce dementia but that meta analysis of the study data combined with other data suggested that further study could be warranted.[39]

Brain-derived neurotrophic factor (BDNF) expression is associated with some dementia types.[40] [41] [42]

A Canadian study found that a lifetime of bilingualism delays the onset of dementia by an average of four years when compared to monolingual patients.[43]

Management

Except for the treatable types listed above, there is no cure to this illness. Cholinesterase inhibitors are often used early in the disease course. Cognitive and behavioral interventions may also be appropriate. Educating and providing emotional support to the caregiver (or carer) is of importance as well (*see also elderly care*).

Pain and dementia

As people age, they experience more health problems, and most health problems associated with aging carry a substantial burden of pain; so, between 25% and 50% of older adults experience persistent pain. Seniors with dementia experience the same prevalence of conditions likely to cause pain as seniors without dementia.[44] Pain is often overlooked in older adults and, when screened for, often poorly assessed, especially among those with dementia since they become incapable of informing others that they're in pain.[44] [45] Beyond the issue of humane care, unrelieved pain has functional implications. Persistent pain can lead to decreased ambulation, depressed mood, sleep disturbances, impaired appetite and exacerbation of cognitive impairment,[45] and pain-related interference with activity is a factor contributing to falls in the elderly.[44] [46]

Although persistent pain in the person with dementia is difficult to communicate, diagnose and treat, failure to address persistent pain has profound functional, psychosocial and quality of life implications for this vulnerable population. Health professionals often lack the skills and usually lack the time needed to recognize, accurately assess and adequately monitor pain in people with dementia.[44] [47] Family members and friends can make a valuable contribution to the care of a person with dementia by learning to recognize and assess their pain. Educational resources (such as the Understand Pain and Dementia [48] tutorial) and observational assessment tools are available.[44] [49] [50]

Medications

Currently, there are no medications that are clinically proven to be preventative or curative of dementia.[51] Although some medications are approved for use in the treatment of dementia, these treat the behavioural and cognitive symptoms of dementia, but have no effect on the underlying pathophysiology.[52]

- Acetylcholinesterase inhibitors: Tacrine (Cognex), donepezil (Aricept), galantamine (Razadyne), and rivastigmine (Exelon) are approved by the United States Food and Drug Administration (FDA) for treatment of dementia induced by Alzheimer's disease. They may be useful for other similar diseases causing dementia such as Parkinsons or vascular dementia.[52] Acetylcholinesterase inhibitors aim to increase the amount of the neurotransmitter acetylcholine, which is deficient in people with dementia.[53] This is done by inhibiting the action of the enzyme acetylcholinesterase, which breaksdown acetylcholine as part of normal brain function.[54] Though these medications are commonly prescribed, in a minority of patients these drugs can cause side effects including bradycardia and syncope.[55]
- N-methyl-D-aspartate (NMDA) receptor blockers: Memantine is marketed under several names by different pharmaceutical companies including: Abixa, Akatinol, Axura, Ebixa, Memox and Namenda.[56] In dementia, NMDA receptors are over-stimulated by glutamate, which creates problems for neurotransmission (and thus cognition) and also leads to damage to neurons through excitotoxicity. Memantine is thought to work by improving the "signal-to-noise" ratio and preventing excitotoxic damage.[57] Hence, due to their differing mechanisms of action memantine and acetylcholinesterase inhibitors can be used in combination with each other.[58] [59]

Off label

- Antidepressant drugs: Depression is frequently associated with dementia and generally worsens the degree of cognitive and behavioral impairment. Antidepressants effectively treat the cognitive and behavioral symptoms of depression in patients with Alzheimer's disease,[60] but evidence for their use in other forms of dementia is weak.[61]
- Anxiolytic drugs: Many patients with dementia experience anxiety symptoms. Although benzodiazepines like diazepam (Valium) have been used for treating anxiety in other situations, they are often avoided because they may increase agitation in persons with dementia and are likely to worsen cognitive problems or are too sedating. Buspirone (Buspar) is often initially tried for mild-to-moderate anxiety. There is little evidence for the effectiveness of benzodiazepines in dementia, whereas there is evidence for the effectivess of antipsychotics (at low doses).[62]
- Selegiline, a drug used primarily in the treatment of Parkinson's disease, appears to slow the development of dementia. Selegiline is thought to act as an antioxidant, preventing free radical damage. However, it also acts as a stimulant, making it difficult to determine whether the delay in onset of dementia symptoms is due to protection from free radicals or to the general elevation of brain activity from the stimulant effect.[63]
- Antipsychotic drugs: Both typical antipsychotics (such as Haloperidol) and atypical antipsychotics such as (risperidone) increase the risk of death in dementia-associated psychosis.[64] This means that any use of

antipsychotic medication for dementia-associated psychosis is off-label and should only be considered after discussing the risks and benefits of treatment with these drugs, and after other treatment modalities have failed. In the UK around 144,000 dementia sufferers are unnecessarily prescribed antipsychotic drugs, around 2000 patients die as a result of taking the drugs each year.[65]

Services

Adult daycare centers as well as special care units in nursing homes often provide specialized care for dementia patients. Adult daycare centers offer supervision, recreation, meals, and limited health care to participants, as well as providing respite for caregivers.

In addition, Home care can provide one-on-one support and care in the home allowing for more individualized attention that is needed as the disease progresses.

While some preliminary studies have found that music therapy may be useful in helping patients with dementia, their quality has been low and no reliable conclusions can be drawn from them.[66]

Nursing people with dementia

Psychiatric nurses can make a distinctive contribution to people's mental health. The four main premises upon which psychiatric nursing is based are:

- The nursing is an interactive, developmental human activity that is more concerned with the future development of the person than the origins.
- The experience of mental distress related to the psychiatric disorder is represented through disturbances or reports of private events that are known only to the person concerned.
- Nurses and the people in care are engaged in a relationship based on mutual influence.
- The experience of psychiatric disorder is translated into problems of everyday living and the nurse notes the human responses to the psychiatric distress, not the disorder.[67]

Feeding tubes

There is little evidence, even after widespread use, that feeding tubes help patients with advanced dementia gain weight, regain strength or function, prevent aspiration pneumonias, or improve quality of life. The risks associated with the use of tubes are not well known.[68]

Epidemiology

Evidence from well-planned, representative epidemiological surveys is scarce in many regions, particularly in low-income countries. However, estimates from 2005 suggest a global dementia prevalence of 24.3 million, with 4.6 million new cases of dementia every year. The number of people affected will double every 20 years to 81.1 million by 2040.[69]

See also

- Aging brain
- Caregiving and dementia
- Montessori-Based Dementia Programming
- Agitation (dementia)
- Cognitive orthotics
- Sundowning (dementia)
- Wandering (dementia)
- Aging movement control

References

[1] http://apps.who.int/classifications/icd10/browse/2010/en#/F00

[2] http://apps.who.int/classifications/icd10/browse/2010/en#/F07

[3] http://www.icd9data.com/getICD9Code.ashx?icd9=290

[4] http://www.icd9data.com/getICD9Code.ashx?icd9=294

[5] http://www.diseasesdatabase.com/ddb29283.htm

[6] http://www.nlm.nih.gov/medlineplus/ency/article/000739.htm

[7] http://www.nlm.nih.gov/cgi/mesh/2011/MB_cgi?field=uid&term=D003704

[8] Fadil, H., Borazanci, A., Haddou, E. A. B.,Yahyaoui, M., Korniychuk, E., Jaffe, S. L., Minagar, A. (2009). "Early Onset Dementia". *International Review of Neurobiology*. International Review of Neurobiology **84**: 245–262. doi:10.1016/S0074-7742(09)00413-9. ISBN 9780123748331. PMID 19501722.

[9] "Dementia definition" (http://www.mdguidelines.com/dementia/definition). *MDGuidelines*. Reed Group. . Retrieved 2009-06-04.

[10] Gleason OC (March 2003). "Delirium" (http://www.aafp.org/afp/20030301/1027.html). *American Family Physician* **67** (5): 1027–34. PMID 12643363. .

[11] Berrios GE (November 1987). "Dementia during the seventeenth and eighteenth centuries: a conceptual history". *Psychological Medicine* **17** (4): 829–37. doi:10.1017/S0033291700000623. PMID 3324141.

[12] Kolata, Gina (June 17, 2010). "Drug Trials Test Bold Plan to Slow Alzheimer's" (http://www.nytimes.com/2010/07/17/health/research/17drug.html). *The New York Times*. . Retrieved June 17, 2010.

[13] (http://archneur.ama-assn.org/cgi/content/summary/33/4/217).

[14] Calleo J, Stanley M (2008). "Anxiety Disorders in Later Life Differentiated Diagnosis and Treatment Strategies" (http://www.psychiatrictimes.com/display/article/10168/1166976). *Psychiatric Times* **25** (8). .

[15] Shub, Denis; Kunik, Mark E (April 16, 2009). "Psychiatric Comorbidity in Persons With Dementia: Assessment and Treatment Strategies" (http://www.psychiatrictimes.com/alzheimer-dementia/article/10168/1403050). *Psychiatric Times* **26** (4). .

[16] "Drivers with dementia a growing problem, MDs warn" (http://www.cbc.ca/health/story/2007/09/19/drivers-dementia.html?ref=rss). CBC News, Canada. September 19, 2007. .

[17] Gelder, Mayou, Geddes (2005). Psychiatry. (Pg 141). New York, NY: Oxford University Press Inc.

[18] Neuropathology Group. Medical Research Council Cognitive Function and Aging Study (2001). "Pathological correlates of late-onset dementia in a multicentre, community-based population in England and Wales. Neuropathology Group of the Medical Research Council Cognitive Function and Ageing Study (MRC CFAS)". *Lancet* **357** (9251): 169–75. doi:10.1016/S0140-6736(00)03589-3. PMID 11213093.

[19] Wakisaka Y et al. (2003). "Age-associated prevalence and risk factors of Lewy body pathology in a general population: the Hisayama study". *Acta Neuropathol* **106** (4): 374–82. doi:10.1007/s00401-003-0750-x. PMID 12904992.

[20] White L et al. (2002). "Cerebrovascular pathology and dementia in autopsied Honolulu-Asia Aging Study participants". *Ann N Y Acad Sci* **977** (9): 9–23. doi:10.1111/j.1749-6632.2002.tb04794.x. PMID 12480729.

[21] Ratnavalli E et al. (2002). "The prevalence of frontotemporal dementia". *Neurology* **58** (11): 1615–21. PMID 12058088.

[22] McKee A et al. (2009). "Chronic Traumatic Encephalopathy in Athletes: Progressive Tauopathy following Repetitive Head Injury". *J Neuropathol Exp Neurol* **68** (7): 709–735. doi:10.1097/NEN.0b013e3181a9d503. PMC 2945234. PMID 19535999.

[23] Galvin JE et al. (2006). "Clinical phenotype of Parkinson disease dementia". *Neurology* **67** (9): 1605–11. doi:10.1212/01.wnl.0000242630.52203.8f. PMID 17101891.

[24] Gibbons D et al.. "Porphyria and dementia: a case report" (http://www.ijpm.org/content/pdf/195/Dementia.pdf). *Ir J Psych Med* **20** (3): 96–99. .

[25] Lamont P (2004). "Cognitive Decline in a Young Adult with Pre-Existent Developmental Delay – What the Adult Neurologist Needs to Know" (http://pn.bmj.com/cgi/content/abstract/4/2/70). *Practical Neurology* **4** (2): 70–87. doi:10.1111/j.1474-7766.2004.02-206.x. .

[26] Boustani, M; Peterson, B; Hanson, L; Harris, R; & Lohr, K; U.S. Preventive Services Task Force (3 June 2003). "Screening for dementia in primary care: a summary of the evidence for the U.S. Preventive Services Task Force" (http://www.annals.org/cgi/content/full/138/11/927). *Ann Intern Med* **138** (11): 927–37. PMID 12779304. .

[27] Cullen B, O'Neill B, Evans JJ, Coen RF, Lawlor BA (August 2007). "A review of screening tests for cognitive impairment". *Journal of Neurology, Neurosurgery, and Psychiatry* **78** (8): 790–9. doi:10.1136/jnnp.2006.095414. PMC 2117747. PMID 17178826.

[28] Teng EL, Chui HC (August 1987). "The Modified Mini-Mental State (3MS) examination". *The Journal of Clinical Psychiatry* **48** (8): 314–8. PMID 3611032.

[29] Teng EL, Hasegawa K, Homma A, et al. (1994). "The Cognitive Abilities Screening Instrument (CASI): a practical test for cross-cultural epidemiological studies of dementia". *International Psychogeriatrics / IPA* **6** (1): 45–58; discussion 62. doi:10.1017/S1041610294001602. PMID 8054493.

[30] Royall, D; Cordes, J.; Polk, M. (1998). "CLOX: an executive clock drawing task" (http://jnnp.bmj.com/cgi/content/full/64/5/588). *J Neurol Neurosurg Psychiatry* **64** (5): 588–94. doi:10.1136/jnnp.64.5.588. PMC 2170069. PMID 9598672. .

[31] Sager MA, Hermann BP, La Rue A, Woodard JL (October 2006). "Screening for dementia in community-based memory clinics" (http://www.wisconsinmedicalsociety.org/_WMS/publications/wmj/issues/wmj_v105n7/sager.pdf) (PDF). *WMJ: Official Publication of the State Medical Society of Wisconsin* **105** (7): 25–9. PMID 17163083. .

[32] Fleisher, A; Sowell, B; Taylor, C; Gamst, A; Petersen, R; Thal, L; Alzheimer's Disease Cooperative Study (2007). "Clinical predictors of progression to Alzheimer disease in amnestic mild cognitive impairment". *Neurology* **68** (19): 1588–95. doi:10.1212/01.wnl.0000258542.58725.4c. PMID 17287448.

[33] Karlawish, J & Clark, C (2003). "Diagnostic evaluation of elderly patients with mild memory problems" (http://www.annals.org/cgi/content/full/138/5/411). *Ann Intern Med* **138** (5): 411–9. PMID 12614094. .

[34] Jorm AF (September 2004). "The Informant Questionnaire on cognitive decline in the elderly (IQCODE): a review". *International Psychogeriatrics / IPA* **16** (3): 275–93. doi:10.1017/S1041610204000390. PMID 15559753.

[35] Bonte, FJ; Harris TS, Hynan LS, Bigio EH, White CL 3rd (July 2006). "Tc-99m HMPAO SPECT in the differential diagnosis of the dementias with histopathologic confirmation". *Clinical Nuclear Medicine* **31** (7): 376–8. doi:10.1097/01.rlu.0000222736.81365.63. PMID 16785801.

[36] Dougall, NJ; Bruggink S, Ebmeier KP (Nov-December 2004). "Systematic review of the diagnostic accuracy of 99mTc-HMPAO-SPECT in dementia". *The American Journal of Geriatric Psychiatry* **12** (6): 554–70. doi:10.1176/appi.ajgp.12.6.554. PMID 15545324.

[37] Abella HA (June 16, 2009). "Report from SNM: PET imaging of brain chemistry bolsters characterization of dementias" (http://www.diagnosticimaging.com/imaging-trends-advances/cardiovascular-imaging/article/113619/1423022). *Diagnostic Imaging*. .

[38] (http://www.time.com/time/health/article/0,8599,1623739,00.html)

> "It is... possible that moderate lifestyles in general, which obviously vary according to different cultural environments, protect from cognitive impairment. Thus it may not be the direct effect of alcohol or specific substances in alcoholic drinks that provide the protection."

[39] Hyvet, investigators; Burch; Fletcher; Bulpitt (August 2008). "Incident dementia and blood pressure lowering in the Hypertension in the Very Elderly Trial cognitive function assessment (HYVET-COG): a double-blind, placebo controlled trial". *Lancet Neurol* **7** (8): 683–9. doi:10.1016/S1474-4422(08)70143-1. PMID 18614402.

[40] Hu, Y; Russek, SJ (2008). "BDNF and the diseased nervous system: a delicate balance between adaptive and pathological processes of gene regulation". *Journal of neurochemistry* **105** (1): 1–17. doi:10.1111/j.1471-4159.2008.05237.x. PMID 18208542.

[41] Schindowski, K; Belarbi, K; Buée, L (2008). "Neurotrophic factors in Alzheimer's disease: role of axonal transport". *Genes, Brain and Behavior* **7** (Suppl 1): 43–56. doi:10.1111/j.1601-183X.2007.00378.x. PMC 2228393. PMID 18184369.

[42] Tapia-Arancibia, L; Aliaga, E; Silhol, M; Arancibia, S (2008). "New insights into brain BDNF function in normal aging and Alzheimer disease". *Brain research reviews* **59** (1): 201–20. doi:10.1016/j.brainresrev.2008.07.007. PMID 18708092.

[43] "Bilingualism Has Protective Effect In Delaying Onset Of Dementia By Four Years, Canadian Study Shows" (http://www.medicalnewstoday.com/medicalnews.php?newsid=60646). Medical News Today. 2007-01-11. . Retrieved 2007-01-16.

[44] Hadjistavropoulos, T et al.; Herr, K; Turk, DC; Fine, PG; Dworkin, RH; Helme, R; Jackson, K; Parmelee, PA et al. (2007). "An interdisciplinary expert consensus statement on assessment of pain in older persons". *Clinical Journal of Pain* **23** (1 suppl): S1–43. doi:10.1097/AJP.0b013e31802be869. PMID 17179836.

[45] Shega, J; Emanuel, L; Vargish, L; Levine, S.K.; Bursch, H; Herr, K; Karp, J.F.; Weiner, D.K. (2007). "Pain in persons with dementia: complex, common, and challenging". *Journal of Pain* **8** (5): 373–8. doi:10.1016/j.jpain.2007.03.003. PMID 17485039.

[46] Blyth, F; Cumming, M.R.; Mitchell, P; Wang, J.J. (2007). "Pain and falls in older people" (http://www.ncbi.nlm.nih.gov/pubmed/17015026?itool=EntrezSystem2.PEntrez.Pubmed.Pubmed_ResultsPanel.Pubmed_RVDocSum&ordinalpos=8). *European Journal of Pain* **11** (5): 564–71. doi:10.1016/j.ejpain.2006.08.001. PMID 17015026. .

[47] Brown, C. (2009). "Pain, aging and dementia: The crisis is looming, but are we ready?" (http://www.ingentaconnect.com/content/cot/bjot/2009/00000072/00000008/art00007). *British Journal of Occupational Therapy* **72** (8): 371–75. .

[48] http://www.painanddementia.ualberta.ca

[49] Herr, K; Bjoro, K; Decker, S; Wang (2006). "Tools for assessment of pain in nonverbal older adults with dementia: a state-of-the-science review" (http://www.ncbi.nlm.nih.gov/pubmed/16488350). *Journal of pain and symptom management* **31** (2): 170–92. doi:10.1016/j.jpainsymman.2005.07.001. PMID 16488350. .

[50] Stolee, P; Hillier, LM; Esbaugh, et al.; Bol, N; McKellar, L; Gauthier, N (2005). "Instruments for the assessment of pain in older persons with cognitive impairment". *Journal of the American geriatrics society* **53** (2): 319–26. doi:10.1111/j.1532-5415.2005.53121.x. PMID 15673359.

[51] Rafii, M. S. & Aisen, P. S. (2009). "Recent developments in Alzheimer's disease therapeutics" (http://www.biomedcentral.com/1741-7015/7/7). *BMC medicine* **7**: 1–4. doi:10.1186/1741-7015-7-7. .

[52] Lleó A, Greenberg SM, Growdon JH (2006). "Current pharmacotherapy for Alzheimer's disease" (http://arjournals.annualreviews.org/doi/abs/10.1146/annurev.med.57.121304.131442?url_ver=Z39.88-2003&rfr_id=ori:rid:crossref.org&rfr_dat=cr_pub=ncbi.nlm.nih.gov). *Annu. Rev. Med.* **57**: 513–33. doi:10.1146/annurev.med.57.121304.131442. PMID 16409164. .

[53] Lleó A, Greenberg SM, Growdon JH (2006). "Current pharmacotherapy for Alzheimer's disease". *Annu. Rev. Med.* **57**: 513–33. doi:10.1146/annurev.med.57.121304.131442. PMID 16409164.

[54] Bear, M. F., Connors, B. W. & Paradiso, M. A. (2007). "5". *Neuroscience: Exploring The Brain*. Baltimore: Lippincott Williams & Wilkins. p. 119. ISBN 0-7817-6003-8.

[55] Gill S. S., Anderson, G. M., Fischer, H.D., Li, P., Normand, S. T. & Rochon, P. A. (2009). "Syncope and its consequences in patients with dementia receiving cholinesterase inhibitors: A population-based cohort study". *Archives of Internal Medicine* **169** (9): 867–873. doi:10.1001/archinternmed.2009.43. PMID 19433698.

[56] Plath, N., Ledrup, L., Larsen P. H. & Redrobe, J. P., Niels; Lerdrup, Linda; Larsen, Peter Hjørringgaard; Redrobe, John Paul (2011). "Can small molecules provide truly effective enhancement of cognition? Current achievements and future directions". *Expert Opinion on Investigational Drugs* **20** (6): 795–811. doi:10.1517/13543784.2011.574612. PMID 21510828.

[57] Parsons, C. G., Stoffler, A. & Danysz, W., Chris G.; Stöffler, Albrecht; Danysz, Wojciech (2007). "Memantine: A NMDA receptor antagonist that improves memory by restoration of homeostasis in the glutamatergic system - too little activation is bad, too much is even worse". *Neuropharmacology* **53** (6): 699–723. doi:10.1016/j.neuropharm.2007.07.013. PMID 17904591.

[58] Raina P, Santaguida P, Ismaila A, et al. (March 2008). "Effectiveness of cholinesterase inhibitors and memantine for treating dementia: evidence review for a clinical practice guideline" (http://www.annals.org/cgi/content/full/148/5/379). *Annals of Internal Medicine* **148** (5): 379–97. PMID 18316756. .

[59] Atri A, Shaughnessy LW, Locascio JJ, Growdon JH (2008). "Long-term Course and Effectiveness of Combination Therapy in Alzheimer's Disease". *Alzheimer Disease and Associated Disorders* **22** (3): 209–21. doi:10.1097/WAD.0b013e31816653bc. PMC 2718545. PMID 18580597.

[60] Thompson S, Herrmann N, Rapoport MJ, Lanctôt KL (April 2007). "Efficacy and safety of antidepressants for treatment of depression in Alzheimer's disease: a metaanalysis" (http://publications.cpa-apc.org/media.php?mid=586&xwm=true) (PDF). *Canadian Journal of Psychiatry* **52** (4): 248–55. PMID 17500306. .

[61] Bains J, Birks JS, Dening TR (2002). Dening, Tom. ed. "The efficacy of antidepressants in the treatment of depression in dementia". *Cochrane Database of Systematic Reviews* (4): CD003944. doi:10.1002/14651858.CD003944. PMID 12519625.

[62] Lolk A, Gulmann NC (2006). "[Psychopharmacological treatment of behavioral and psychological symptoms in dementia]" (in Danish). *Ugeskr Laeg* **168** (40): 3429–32. PMID 17032610.

[63] Riederer P, Lachenmayer L (November 2003). "Selegiline's neuroprotective capacity revisited". *Journal of Neural Transmission* **110** (11): 1273–8. doi:10.1007/s00702-003-0083-x. PMID 14628191.

[64] "FDA MedWatch - 2008 Safety Alerts for Human Medical Products" (http://www.fda.gov/medwatch/safety/2008/safety08.htm#Antipsychotics). *FDA*. .

[65] Bowcott, Owen (2009-11-12). "Chemical restraints killing dementia patients" (http://www.guardian.co.uk/society/2009/nov/12/anti-psychotic-drugs-kill-dementia-patients). London: Guardian. . Retrieved 2010-05-01.

[66] Vink AC, Bruinsma MS, Scholten RJPM; (Dementia and Cognitive Improvement Group) (2003). "Music therapy for people with dementia". *Cochrane Database of Systematic Reviews* (4): CD003477.pub2 (Orig. rev.). doi:10.1002/14651858.CD003477.pub2. PMID 15266489.

[67] Barker, P. (2003). Psychiatric and Mental Health Nursing *The craft of caring*. New York, NY: Oxford University Press Inc.

[68] Sampson EL, Candy B, Jones L; (Dementia and Cognitive Improvement Group) (2009 Apr 15). "Enteral tube feeding for older people with advanced dementia". *Cochrane Database of Systematic Reviews* (2): CD007209.pub2 (Orig. rev.). doi:10.1002/14651858.CD007209.pub2.

[69] Ferri, CP; Prince, M, Brayne, C, Brodaty, H, Fratiglioni, L, Ganguli, M, Hall, K, Hasegawa, K, Hendrie, H, Huang, Y, Jorm, A, Mathers, C, Menezes, PR, Rimmer, E, Scazufca, M, Alzheimer's Disease, International (2005-12-17). "Global prevalence of dementia: a Delphi consensus study". *Lancet* **366** (9503): 2112–7. doi:10.1016/S0140-6736(05)67889-0. PMC 2850264. PMID 16360788.

External links

- BBC Headroom: (http://www.bbc.co.uk/headroom/mental_health/alzheimers_and_dementia.shtml) Living with Dementia
- The Dementia Centre (http://www.dementiacentre.com) – Information provided by PSS (Personal Services Society). Provides information and support to people with dementia, their carers, and health professionals.
- Alzheimer's Research Trust – What is dementia? (http://www.alzheimers-research.org.uk/info/dementia/) – Information produced by the Alzheimer's Research Trust including statistics.
- Alzheimer's Society – About dementia (http://www.alzheimers.org.uk/site/scripts/documents.php?categoryID=200120) – Information produced by the Alzheimer's Society including factsheets and support.
- The Dementia Services Development Centre, University of Stirling (http://www.dementia.stir.ac.uk)
- Dementia tutorial for U.K. practitioners by the Alzheimer's Society (http://www.ehr.chime.ucl.ac.uk/display/demcare/Home)
- Understanding Dementia: a primer of diagnosis and management (http://www.dementiaguide.ca/aboutdementia/understanding/)
- AlzOnline (http://alzonline.phhp.ufl.edu) – AlzOnline provides education, information, and support to persons caring for someone with Alzheimer's disease or a related memory problem.
- Medicinenet (http://www.medicinenet.com/dementia/article.htm)
- Understand Pain and Dementia tutorial (http://www.painanddementia.ualberta.ca) from the Occupational Therapy Department at the University of Alberta
- Help Dementia Uk (http://helpdementia.org.uk/)
- Concise Guidelines to Better Practice (http://www.britishpainsociety.org/book_pain_older_people.pdf) The Assessment of Pain in Older Person – British Pain Society (2007)
- Dementia care map (http://eng.mapofmedicine.com/evidence/map/dementia1.html) Map of Medicine, Updated 29 October 2010
- *Dementia* (http://www.gpnotebook.co.uk/simplepage.cfm?ID=-1650851840) at GPnotebook
- *Dementia* (http://www.emedicinehealth.com/dementia_overview/article_em.htm) at eMedicineHealth
- Merck Geriatrics *5-40a* (http://www.merck.com/mrkshared/mmg/sec5/ch40/ch40a.jsp)
- Does Alcohol Slow Dementia? (http://www.time.com/time/health/article/0,8599,1623739,00.html)

Safety_Confirmation

Safety Confirmation is a way of determining each day whether someone who lives alone is safe. All the person has to do is to press, before a time agreed with him or her, an 'I am okay' button on a special landline or mobile phone handset that can also be used normally to make calls. The button-press is transmitted to a monitoring centre and managed automatically. A follow-up system is initiated if a user fails to confirm that they are okay. If the button is not pressed by the agreed time it can be taken as a passive request for contact.

By the application of 'lean' design, the process of Safety Confirmation is conceptually simple[1] , especially for people who use it but, as it has to be highly dependable and work reliably over different providers' phone networks, the technology that runs it is complex.

Safety Confirmation was invented and brought to market by James Batchelor (May 28th, 1977, Yorkshire, England), a British technology entrepreneur and inventor who created it when he spotted the shortcomings of the predominant paradigm of personal safety alarms (also known as: community alarms; pendant alarms; autodialer alarms; medical alerts or personal emergency response systems (PERS)) after his grandmother fell.

Conventionally, people who may be prone to falling or medical emergencies are provided with a button to press if they need help, which raises a call to a monitoring centre (as in the famous US TV advertisement "Help, I've Fallen and I Can't Get up"). A study reported in 2010 found that only 8% of people with pendant alarms wore them at all times and that two-thirds had never used them.[2]

By reversing the conventional paradigm Safety Confirmation provides reassurance for carers and avoids the situation where a person with a conventional alarm system is unable or unwilling to use it. The supplier[3] reports that sudden changes in a daily pattern of the 'I am OK' button presses can be indicative of changes in general well being and, as the system is so simple to use, it functions as a cognitive test with deteriorating performance indicating that the user is developing further needs.

Safety Confirmation has been on sale in the UK since 2005[4] and is used by local councils as part of their preventative telecare strategy.

References

[1] Poplar HARCA housing provider (http://www.poplarharca.co.uk/News/NEWPOPLARHARCASERVICEHELPSOLDERRESIDENTSSTAYSAFEANDINDEPENDENT)

[2] Telecare Aware (http://www.telecareaware.com/index.php/pendant-alarms-users-dont-use.html)

[3] Alertacall (http://www.alertacall.com/)

[4] Yorkshire Forward (http://www.yorkshire-forward.com/news-events/news/local-news/new-telephone-system-to-check-on-loved)

External links

- Yorkshire Post (http://www.yorkshirepost.co.uk/businessnews/Idea-that-came-blowing-in.1215166.jp)
- Craven Herald: Source of inspiration for Safety Confirmation (http://www.cravenherald.co.uk/archive/2005/10/07/Bradford+District+Archive/8083252.Grandma_inspires_new_safety_invention/)

Telemedicine

Telemedicine is the use of telecommunication and information technologies in order to provide clinical health care at a distance. It helps eliminate distance barriers and can improve access to medical services that would often not be consistently available in distant rural communities. It is also used to save lives in critical care and emergency situations.

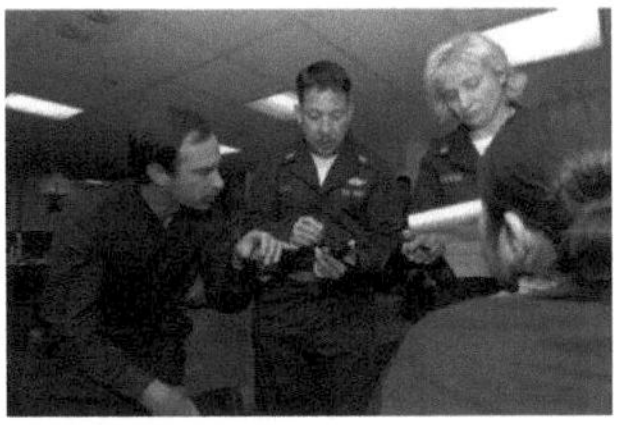

U.S. Navy medical staff being trained in the use of handheld telemedical devices (2006).

Although there were distant precursors to telemedicine, it is essentially a product of 20th century telecommunication and information technologies. These technologies permit communications between patient and medical staff with both convenience and fidelity, as well as the transmission of medical, imaging and heath informatics data from one site to another.

Early forms of telemedicine achieved with telephone and radio have been supplemented with videotelephony, advanced diagnostic methods supported by distributed client/server applications, and additionally with telemedical devices to support in-home care.[1]

Disambiguation

Other expressions similar to telemedicine are the terms "telehealth" and "eHealth", which are frequently used to denote broader definitions of remote healthcare not always involving active clinical treatments.[2] Telehealth and eHealth are at times incorrectly interchanged with telemedicine. Like the terms "medicine" and "health care", telemedicine often refers only to the provision of clinical services while the term telehealth can refer to clinical and non-clinical services involving medical education, administration, and research.[3]

The term eHealth is often used, particularly in the U.K. and Europe, as an umbrella term that includes telehealth, electronic medical records, and other components of health information technology.

Early precursors

In its early manifestations, African villagers used smoke signals to warn people to stay away from the village in case of serious disease.[4] [5] In the early 1900s, people living in remote areas of Australia used two-way radios, powered by a dynamo driven by a set of bicycle pedals, to communicate with the Royal Flying Doctor Service of Australia.

Types of telemedicine

Categories

Telemedicine can be broken into three main categories: store-and-forward, remote monitoring and (real-time) interactive services.

Store-and-forward telemedicine involves acquiring medical data (like medical images, biosignals etc.) and then transmitting this data to a doctor or medical specialist at a convenient time for assessment offline.[2] It does not require the presence of both parties at the same time.[1] Dermatology (cf: teledermatology), radiology, and pathology are common specialties that are conducive to asynchronous telemedicine. A properly structured medical record preferably in electronic form should be a component of this transfer. A key difference between traditional in-person patient meetings and telemedicine encounters is the omission of an actual physical examination and history. The 'store-and-forward' process requires the clinician to rely on a history report and audio/video information in lieu of a physical examination.

Remote monitoring, also known as self-monitoring or testing, enables medical professionals to monitor a patient remotely using various technological devices. This method is primarily used for managing chronic diseases or specific conditions, such as heart disease, diabetes mellitus, or asthma. These services can provide comparable health outcomes to traditional in-person patient encounters, supply greater satisfaction to patients, and may be cost-effective.

Interactive telemedicine services provide real-time interactions between patient and provider, to include phone conversations, online communication and home visits.[1] Many activities such as history review, physical examination, psychiatric evaluations and ophthalmology assessments can be conducted comparably to those done in traditional face-to-face visits. In addition, "clinician-interactive" telemedicine services may be less costly than in-person clinical visit

Emergency telemedicine

Common daily emergency telemedicine is performed by SAMU Regulator Physicians in France, Spain, Chile, Brazil. Aircraft and maritime emergencies are also handled by SAMU centres in Paris, Lisbon and Toulouse.[6]

General health care delivery

Benefits and uses

Telemedicine can be extremely beneficial for people living in isolated communities and remote regions and is currently being applied in virtually all medical domains. Patients who live in such areas can be seen by a doctor or specialist, who can provide an accurate and complete examination, while the patient may not have to travel or wait the normal distances or times like those from conventional hospital or GP visits. Recent developments in mobile collaboration technology with the use of hand-held mobile devices allow healthcare professionals in multiple locations the ability to view, discuss and assess patient issues as if they were in the same room.[7]

Telemedicine can be used as a teaching tool, by which experienced medical staff can observe, show and instruct medical staff in another location, more effective or faster examination techniques. It improved access to healthcare for patients in remote locations. "Telemedicine has been shown to reduce the cost of healthcare and increase efficiency through better management of chronic diseases,shared health professional staffing, reduced travel times, and fewer or shorter hospital stays." Several studies have documented increase patient satisfaction of telemedicine over past fifteen years.[8]

The first interactive telemedicine system, operating over standard telephone lines, for remotely diagnosing and treating patients requiring cardiac resuscitation (defibrillation) was developed and marketed by MedPhone Corporation in 1989 under the leadership of its president and founder, S.Eric Wachtel. A year later the company introduced a mobile cellular version, the MDphone. Twelve hospitals in the U.S. served as receiving and treatment centers.[9]

Telemonitoring is a medical practice that involves remotely monitoring patients who are not at the same location as the health care provider. In general, a patient will have a number of monitoring devices at home, and the results of these devices will be transmitted via telephone to the health care provider. Telemonitoring is a convenient way for patients to avoid travel and to perform some of the more basic work of healthcare for themselves.

In addition to objective technological monitoring, most telemonitoring programs include subjective questioning regarding the patient's health and comfort. This questioning can take place automatically over the phone, or telemonitoring software can help keep the patient in touch with the health care provider. The provider can then make decisions about the patient's treatment based on a combination of subjective and objective information similar to what would be revealed during an on-site appointment.

Some of the more common things that telemonitoring devices keep track of include blood pressure, heart rate, weight, blood glucose, and hemoglobin. Telemonitoring is capable of providing information about any vital signs, as long as the patient has the necessary monitoring equipment at his or her location. Depending on the severity of the patient's condition, the provider may check these statistics on a daily or weekly basis to determine the best course of treatment.

The first Ayurvedic telemedicine center was established in India in 2007 by Partap Chauhan, an Indian Ayurvedic doctor and the Director of Jiva Ayurveda.

Monitoring a patient at home using known devices like blood pressure monitors and transferring the information to a caregiver is a fast growing emerging service. These remote monitoring solutions have a focus on current high morbidity chronic diseases and are mainly deployed for the First World. In developing countries a new way of practicing telemedicine is emerging better known as Primary Remote Diagnostic Visits, whereby a doctor uses devices to remotely examine and treat a patient. This new technology and principle of practicing medicine holds significant promise of improving on major health care delivery problems, in for instance, Southern Africa, because Primary Remote Diagnostic Consultations not only monitors an already diagnosed chronic disease, but has the promise to diagnose and manage the diseases patients will typically visit a general practitioner for.

Telenursing

Telenursing refers to the use of telecommunications and information technology in order to provide nursing services in health care whenever a large physical distance exists between patient and nurse, or between any number of nurses. As a field it is part of telehealth, and has many points of contacts with other medical and non-medical applications, such as telediagnosis, teleconsultation, telemonitoring, etc.

Telenursing is achieving significant growth rates in many countries due to several factors: the preoccupation in reducing the costs of health care, an increase in the number of aging and chronically ill population, and the increase in coverage of health care to distant, rural, small or sparsely populated regions. Among its benefits, telenursing may help solve increasing shortages of nurses; to reduce distances and save travel time, and to keep patients out of hospital. A greater degree of job satisfaction has been registered among telenurses.[10]

Telepharmacy

Telepharmacy is another growing trend for providing pharmaceutical care to patients at remote locations where they may not have physical contact with pharmacists. It encompasses drug therapy monitoring, patient counseling, prior authorization, refill authorization, monitoring formulary compliance with the aid of teleconferencing or videoconferencing. In addition, video-conferencing is vastly utilized in pharmacy for other purposes, such as providing education, training, and performing several management functions.[11]

A notable telepharmacy program is in the United States, conducted at a federally qualified community health center, Community Health Association of Spokane (CHAS) in 2001, which allowed the low cost medication dispensing under federal government's program. This program utilized videotelephony for dispensing medication and patient counseling at six urban and rural clinics. There were one base pharmacy and five remote clinics in several areas of Spokane, Washington under the telepharmacy program at CHAS. "The base pharmacy provided traditional pharmacy study to the clients at Valley clinic and served as the hub pharmacy for the other remote clinics."

The remote site dispensing and patient education process was described as follows: once the prescription is sent from the remote clinics to the base pharmacy, the pharmacist verifies the hard copy and enters the order. The label is also generated simultaneously, and the label queue is transmitted to the remote site. When the label queue appears on the medication dispensing cabinet known as ADDS, the authorized person can access the medicine from ADDS followed by medication barcode scanning, and the printing and scanning of labels. Once those steps are done, the remote site personnel are connected to the pharmacist at base pharmacy via videoconferencing for medication verification and patient counseling.[12]

In recent time, the U.S. Navy Bureau of Medicine took a significant step in advancing telepharmacy worldwide. The telepharmacy program was piloted in 2006 "in the regions served by Naval Hospital Pensacola, Florida, and Naval

Hospital Bremerton, Washington." Starting from March 2010, the Navy expanded its telepharmacy system to more sites throughout the world. According to Navy Lieutenant Justin Eubanks at Navy Hospital Pensacola, Florida, telepharmacy would be initiated at more than 100 Navy sites covering four continents by the end of 2010.[13]

Telerehabilitation

Telerehabilitation (or *e-rehabilitation*[14] [15]) is the delivery of rehabilitation services over telecommunication networks and the Internet. Most types of services fall into two categories: clinical assessment (the patient's functional abilities in his or her environment), and clinical therapy. Some fields of rehabilitation practice that have explored telerehabilitation are: neuropsychology, speech-language pathology, audiology, occupational therapy, and physical therapy. Telerehabilitation can deliver therapy to people who cannot travel to a clinic because the patient has a disability or because of travel time. Telerehabilitation also allows experts in rehabilitation to engage in a clinical consultation at a distance.

Most telerehabilitation is highly visual. As of 2006 the most commonly used modalities are via webcams, videoconferencing, phone lines, videophones and webpages containing rich Internet applications. The visual nature of telerehabilitation technology limits the types of rehabilitation services that can be provided. It is most widely used for neuropsychological rehabilitation; fitting of rehabilitation equipment such as wheelchairs, braces or artificial limbs; and in speech-language pathology. Rich internet applications for neuropsychological rehabilitation (aka cognitive rehabilitation) of cognitive impairment (from many etiologies) was first introduced in 2001. This endeavor has recently (2006) expanded as a teletherapy application for cognitive skills enhancement programs for school children. Tele-audiology (hearing assessments) is a growing application. As of 2006, telerehabilitation in the practice of occupational therapy and physical therapy are very limited, perhaps because these two disciplines are more “hands on".

Two important areas of telerehabilitation research are (1) demonstrating equivalence of assessment and therapy to in-person assessment and therapy, and (2) building new data collection systems to digitize information that a therapist can use in practice. Ground-breaking research in telehaptics (the sense of touch) and virtual reality may broaden the scope of telerehabilitation practice, in the future.

In the United States, the National Institute on Disability and Rehabilitation Research's (NIDRR) [16] supports research and the development of telerehabilitation. NIDRR's grantees include the "Rehabilitation Engineering and Research Center" (RERC) at the University of Pittsburgh, the Rehabilitation Institute of Chicago, the State University of New York at Buffalo, and the National Rehabilitation Hospital in Washington DC. Other federal funders of research are the Veterans Administration, the Health Services Research Administration in the US Department of Health and Human Services, and the Department of Defense. Outside the United States, excellent research is conducted in Australia and Europe.

As of 2006, only a few health insurers in the United States will reimburse for telerehabilitation services. If the research shows that teleassessments and teletherapy are equivalent to clinical encounters, it is more likely that insurers and Medicare will cover telerehabilitation services.

Specialist care delivery

Telemedicine can facilitate specialty care delivered by primary care physicians according to a controlled study of the treatment of hepatitis C.[17] Various specialties are contributing to telemedicine, in varying degrees.

Telecardiology

ECGs, or electrocardiographs, can be transmitted using telephone and wireless. Willem Einthoven, the inventor of the ECG, actually did tests with transmission of ECG via telephone lines. This was because the hospital did not allow him to move patients outside the hospital to his laboratory for testing of his new device. In 1906 Einthoven came up with a way to transmit the data from the hospital directly to his lab.[18]

Teletransmission of ECG using methods indigenous to Asia

One of the oldest known telecardiology systems for teletransmissions of ECGs was established in Gwalior, India in 1975 at GR Medical college by Dr. Ajai Shanker, Dr. S. Makhija, P.K. Mantri using an indegenous technique for the first time in India.

This system enabled wireless transmission of ECG from the moving ICU van or the patients home to the central station in ICU of the department of Medicine. Transmission using wireless was done using frequency modulation which eliminated noise. Transmission was also done through telephone lines. The ECG output was connected to the telephone input using a modulator which converted ECG into high frequency sound. At the other end a demodulator reconverted the sound into ECG with a good gain accuracy. The ECG was converted to sound waves with a frequency varying from 500 Hz to 2500 Hz with 1500 Hz at baseline.

This system was also used to monitor patients with pacemakers in remote areas. The central control unit at the ICU was able to correctly interpret arrhythmia. This technique helped medical aid reach in remote areas.[19]

In addition, electronic stethoscopes can be used as recording devices, which is helpful for purposes of telecardiology.

In Pakistan three pilot projects in telemedicine was initiated by the Ministry of IT & Telecom, Government of Pakistan (MoIT) through the Electronic Government Directorate in collaboration with Oratier Technologies (a pioneer company within Pakistan dealing with healthcare and HMIS) and PakDataCom (a bandwidth provider). Three hub stations through were linked via the Pak Sat-I communications satellite, and four districts were linked with another hub. A 312 Kb link was also established with remote sites and 1 Mbit/s bandwidth was provided at each hub. Three hubs were established: the Mayo Hospital (the largest hospital in Asia), JPMC Karachi and Holy Family Rawalpindi. These 12 remote sites were connected and on average of 1,500 patients being treated per month per hub. The project was still running smoothly after two years.[20]

Telepsychiatry

Telepsychiatry, another aspect of telemedicine, also utilizes videoconferencing for patients residing in underserved areas to access psychiatric services. It offers wide range of services to the patients and providers, such as consultation between the psychiatrists, educational clinical program, diagnosis and assessment, medication therapy management, etc.

The following are some of the model programs and projects which are undergoing for implementation of telepsychiatry in rural areas in the US.

1. University of Colorado Health Sciences Center (UCHSC) supports two programs for American Indian and Alaskan Native populations

    a. The Center for Native American Telehealth and Tele-education (CNATT) and

    b. Telemental Health Treatment for American Indian Veterans with Posttraumatic Stress Disorder (PTSD)

2. Military Psychiatry, Walter Reed Army Medical Center.

Links for several sites related to telemedicine, telepsychiatry policy, guidelines, and networking are available at the website for the American Psychiatric Association.[21]

Teleradiology

Teleradiology is the ability to send radiographic images (x-rays, CT, MR, PET/CT, SPECT/CT, MG, US...) from one location to another.[22] For this process to be implemented, three essential components are required, an image sending station, a transmission network, and a receiving-image review station. The most typical implementation are two computers connected via the Internet. The computer at the receiving end will need to have a high-quality display screen that has been tested and cleared for clinical purposes. Sometimes the receiving computer will have a printer so that images can be printed for convenience.

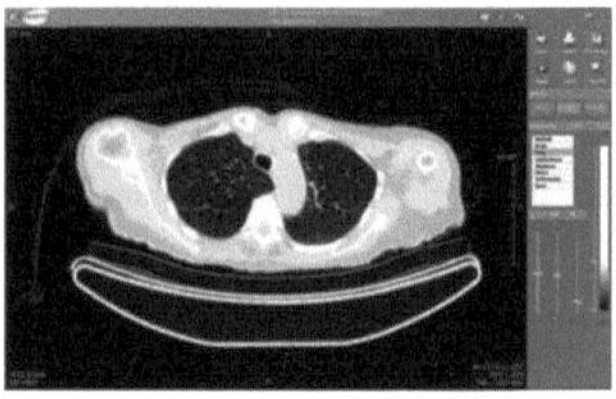

A CT exam displayed through teleradiology

The teleradiology process begins at the image sending station. The radiographic image and a modem or other connection are required for this first step. The image is scanned and then sent via the network connection to the receiving computer.

Today's high-speed broadband based Internet enables the use of new technologies for teleradiology : the image reviewer can now have access to distant servers in order to view an exam. Therefore, they do not need particular workstations to view the images ; a standard Personal Computer (PC) and Digital Subscriber Line (DSL) connection is enough to reach keosys central server. No particular software is necessary on the PC and the images can be reached from wherever in the world.

Teleradiology is the most popular use for telemedicine and accounts for at least 50% of all telemedicine usage.

Telepathology

Telepathology is the practice of pathology at a distance. It uses telecommunications technology to facilitate the transfer of image-rich pathology data between distant locations for the purposes of diagnosis, education, and research.[23] [24] Performance of telepathology requires that a pathologist selects the video images for analysis and the rendering diagnoses. The use of “television microscopy”, the forerunner of telepathology, did not require that a pathologist have physical or virtual “hands-on” involvement is the selection of microscopic fields-of-view for analysis and diagnosis.

A pathologist, Ronald S. Weinstein,M.D., coined the term “telepathology” in 1986. In an editorial in a medical journal, Weinstein outlined the actions that would be needed to create remote pathology diagnostic services.[25] He, and his collaborators, published the first scientific paper on robotic telepathology.[26] Weinstein was also granted the first U.S. patents for robotic telepathology systems and telepathology diagnostic networks.[27] Dr. Weinstein is known to many as the "father of telepathology".[28] In Norway, Eide and Nordrum implemented the first sustainable clinical telepathology service in 1989.[29] This is still in operation, decades later. A number of clinical telepathology services have benefited many thousands of patients in North America, Europe, and Asia.

Telepathology has been successfully used for many applications including the rendering histopathology tissue diagnoses, at a distance, for education, and for research. Although digital pathology imaging, including virtual microscopy, is the mode of choice for telepathology services in developed countries, analog telepathology imaging is still used for patient services in some developing countries.

Teledermatology

Teledermatology is a subspecialty in the medical field of dermatology and probably one of the most common applications of telemedicine and e-health.[30] In teledermatology, telecommunication technologies are used to exchange medical information (concerning skin conditions and tumours of the skin) over a distance using audio, visual and data communication. Applications comprise health care management such as diagnoses, consultation and treatment as well as (continuous) education.[31]

The dermatologists Perednia and Brown were the first to coin the term "teledermatology" in 1995. In a scientific publication, they described the value of a teledermatologic service in a rural area underserved by dermatologists.[32]

Teledentistry

Teledentistry is the use of information technology and telecommunications for dental care, consultation, education, and public awareness in the same manner as telehealth and telemedicine.

Tele-audiology

Tele-audiology is the utilization of telehealth to provide audiological services and may include the full scope of audiological practice.

This term was first used by Dr Gregg Givens in 1999 in reference to a system being developed at East Carolina University in North Carolina, USA. The first Internet audiological test was accomplished in 2000 by Givens, Balch and Keller.

The first Transatlantic teleaudiology test was performed in April 2009 when Dr James Hall tested a patient in South Africa from Dallas.

U.S. licensing and regulatory issues

Restrictive licensure laws in the United States require a practitioner to obtain a full license to deliver telemedicine care across state lines. Typically, states with restrictive licensure laws also have several exceptions (varying from state to state) that may release an out-of-state practitioner from the additional burden of obtaining such a license. A number of States require practitioners who seek compensation to frequently deliver interstate care to acquire a full license.

If a practitioner serves several states, obtaining this license in each state could be an expensive and time-consuming proposition. Even if the practitioner never practices medicine face-to-face with a patient in another state, he/she still must meet a variety of other individual state requirements, including paying substantial licensure fees, passing additional oral and written examinations, and traveling for interviews.

Regulations concerning the practice of telemedicine vary from state to state.[33] Physicians who will be prescribing over the Internet to patients should mandate strict controls on their practice to insure that they stay compliant with the various State Medical Board Regulations concerning Internet Prescribing.[34]

Advanced and experimental services

Telesurgery

Remote surgery (also known as **telesurgery**) is the ability for a doctor to perform surgery on a patient even though they are not physically in the same location. It is a form of telepresence. Remote surgery combines elements of robotics, cutting edge communication technology such as high-speed data connections and elements of management information systems. While the field of robotic surgery is fairly well established, most of these robots are controlled by surgeons at the location of the surgery.

Remote surgery is essentially advanced telecommuting for surgeons, where the physical distance between the surgeon and the patient is immaterial. It promises to allow the expertise of specialized surgeons to be available to patients worldwide, without the need for patients to travel beyond their local hospital.[35]

Enabling technologies

Further information: List of video telecommunication services and product brands

Videotelephony

Videotelephony comprises the technologies for the reception and transmission of audio-video signals by users at different locations, for communication between people in real-time.[36]

At the dawn of the technology, videotelephony also included *image phones* which would exchange still images between units every few seconds over conventional POTS-type telephone lines, essentially the same as slow scan TV systems.

Currently videotelephony is particularly useful to the deaf and speech-impaired who can use them with sign language and also with a video relay service, and well as to those with mobility issues or those who are located in distant places and are in need of telemedical or tele-educational services.

Health information technology

Health information technology (HIT) provides the umbrella framework to describe the comprehensive management of health information across computerized systems and its secure exchange between consumers, providers, government and quality entities, and insurers. Health information technology (HIT) is in general increasingly viewed as the most promising tool for improving the overall quality, safety and efficiency of the health delivery system (Chaudhry et al., 2006). Broad and consistent utilization of HIT will:

- Improve health care quality;
- Prevent medical errors;
- Reduce health care costs;
- Increase administrative efficiencies
- Decrease paperwork; and
- Expand access to affordable care.

Interoperable HIT will improve individual patient care, but it will also bring many public health benefits including:

- Early detection of infectious disease outbreaks around the country;
- Improved tracking of chronic disease management; and
- Evaluation of health care based on value enabled by the collection of de-identified price and quality information that can be compared.

See also

- American Telemedicine Association
- Centre for e-Health
- Connected Health
- eHealth
- List of video telecommunication services and product brands
- Medical device
- mHealth
- Mobile collaboration
- National Rural Health Association

- Ontario Telemedicine Network
- Remote therapy
- Robotic surgery
- Tele-epidemiology
- Telecare
- Telehealth
- Telemental Health
- Telephone triage
- UNESCO Chair in Telemedicine
- Women on Web

References

[1] Sachpazidis, Ilias Image and Medical Data Communication Protocols for Telemedicine and Teleradiology (dissertation) (ftp://82.135.241.67/Articles/article_11.pdf), Department of Computer Science, Technical University of Darmstadt, Germany, 10 July 2008.

[2] American Telemedicine Association. Telemedicine/Telehealth Terminology (http://www.americantelemed.org/files/public/abouttelemedicine/Terminology.pdf), American Telemedicine Association website, Washington, D.C. Retrieved August 21, 2011.

[3] About Telehealth: Telehealth Definition (http://www.coachorg.com/CTF/about_telehealth/what_is_telehealth.htm), Canadian Telehealth Forum. Retrieved from Coach: Canada's Health Teleinformatics Association website on August 21, 2011.

[4] Did You Know? New Insights Into A World That Is Full of Astonishing Stories and Astounding Facts (http://books.google.ca/books?id=4tgqsTknBcUC), Reader's Digest, Reader's Digest Association Limited, 1990, pg.189, ISBN 0276420144, ISBN 9780276420146.

[5] Nakajima, I.; Sastrokusumo, U.; Mishra, S.K.; Komiya, R.; Malik, A.Z.; Tanuma, T. The Asia Pacific Telecommunity's Telemedicine Activities (http://ieeexplore.ieee.org/xpl/freeabs_all.jsp?arnumber=1717870), IEEE Xplore.com website, 17-19 Aug. 2006, pp. 280 - 282, ISBN 0-7803-9704-5, DOI: 10.1109/HEALTH.2006.246471

[6] George R. Schwartz, C. Gene Cayten; George R. Schwartz (editor). Principles and Practice of Emergency Medicine, Volume 2 (http://books.google.ca/books?id=NlZ_aST4_hcC), Lea & Febiger, 1992, pg.3202, ISBN 081211373X, ISBN 9780812113730.

[7] Van't Haaff, Corey (March/April 2009). "Virtually On-sight" (http://www.justforcanadiandoctors.com/pastissues/JFCD2009/JFCD-Mar-Apr2009.pdf). *Just for Canadian Doctors*. pp. 22. .

[8] What Is Telemedicine? (http://www.americantelemed.org/files/public/abouttelemedicine/What_Is_Telemedicine.pdf)

[9] W. John Blyth. "Telecommunications, Concepts, Development, and Management", Second Edition, Glencoe/McCgraw-Hill Company,1990, pp.280-282.

[10] Nurses Happier Using Telecare, Says International Survey (http://www.e-health-insider.com/news/item.cfm?ID=1263), eHealth Insider website, 15 June 2005, retrieved 2009-04-04;

[11] Angaran, DM. "Telemedicine and Telepharmacy: Current Status and Future Implications", American Journal of Health-System Pharmacy, 1999 Jul 15; Vol. 56: 1405-26

[12] Dennis Clifton, G.; Byer, Heather; Heaton, Kristi; Haberman, Deborah J.; and Gill, Harbir. "Provision of Pharmacy Services to Underserved Populations Via Remote Dispensing and Two-Way Videoconferencing." American Journal of Health-System Pharmacy. 2003 Dec 15; Vol. 60:2577-82

[13] Traynor, Kate. "Navy takes Telepharmacy Worldwide", American Journal of Health-System Pharmacy. 2010 Jul 15; Vol. 67:1134-36

[14] *E-health care information systems: an introduction for students and professionals*, John Wiley and Sons, 2005, p. 219, ISBN 9780787966188

[15] Lisa Keaton; Linda L. Pierce; Victoria Steiner; Karen Lance. "An E-rehabilitation Team Helps Caregivers Deal with Stroke" (http://ijahsp.nova.edu/articles/vol2num4/pierce-keaton.htm). *The Internet Journal of Allied Health Sciences and Practice* (Ijahsp.nova.edu) **2.4**. ISSN 1540-580X. . Retrieved 2011-03-26.

[16] http://www.ed.gov/about/offices/list/osers/nidrr/index.html?src=mr

[17] Arora, Sanjeev; Karla Thornton, Glen Murata, Paulina Deming, Summers Kalishman, Denise Dion, Brooke Parish, Thomas Burke, Wesley Pak, Jeffrey Dunkelberg, Martin Kistin, John Brown, Steven Jenkusky, Miriam Komaromy, Clifford Qualls (2011-06). "Outcomes of Treatment for Hepatitis C Virus Infection by Primary Care Providers" (http://www.nejm.org/doi/full/10.1056/NEJMoa1009370). *New England Journal of Medicine*: 110601140030042. doi:10.1056/NEJMoa1009370. ISSN 0028-4793. . Retrieved 2011-06-02.

[18] Telecardiology (http://www.medetel.lu/download/2009/parallel_sessions/presentation/day1/telecardiology_and_tele-ecg_network.pdf).

[19] "Teletransmission of ECG Waveform: An Ingenious Low Priced Technique", Indian Heart Journal, 1982, Vol.34, No.6.

[20] Pakistan telemedicine (http://202.83.164.29/egdsite04/?p=projimpu)

[21] American Psychiatric Association (http://www.psych.org/Departments/HSF/UnderservedClearinghouse/Linkeddocuments/telepsychiatry.aspx)

[22] Kontaxakis, George; Visvikis, Dimitris; Ohl, Roland; Sachpazidis, Ilias; Suarez, Juan Pablo; Selby, Boris Peter; et al.: "Integrated Telemedicine Applications and Services for Oncological Positron Emission Tomography", Oncology Reports, Vol.15: 1091–1100, 2006

[23] Weinstein, RS; Graham, AM; Richter, LC; Barker, GP; Krupinski, EA; Lopez, AM; Yagi, Y; Gilbertson, JR et al. (2009), "Overview of telepathology, virtual microscopy and whole slide imagining: Prospects for the future.", *Hum Pathol* **40**: 1057–1069
[24] Kumar, S (2009), Kumar S, Dunn BE (editors), ed., "Telepathology: An Audit", *In: Telepathology* (Springer-Verlag Berlin Heidelberg): 225–229
[25] Weinstein, RS (1986), "Prospect for telepatholgy (Editorial)", *Hum Pathol* **17**: 443-434
[26] Weinstein, RS; Bloom, KJ (1987), "Telepathology and the networking of pathology diagnostic services.", *Arch Path Lab Med* **111**: 646–652
[27] Kayser, K; Szymas, J; Weinstein (1999), "Telepathology: Telecommunications, Electronic Education and Publication in Pathology", *Springer, NY*: 1–186
[28] http://www.union.edu/N/DS/s.php?s=8942
[29] Nordrum, I; Engum, B; Rinde, E`; *et al* (1991), "Remote frozen section service: A telepathology project to northern Norway.", *Hum Pathol* **1991**: 514–518
[30] http://www.atmeda.org/icot/sigtelederm.htm
[31] Wooton et al. 2005 Roy soc of med press; Wurm et al. 2007 JDDG; Burg et al. 2005 Teledermatology
[32] Perednia, Brown 1995 Bull Med Libr Assoc
[33] Information Provided for Physicians: Doctors Seeking a Medical Licensing Service (http://www.medlicense.com/telemedicine_license.html), MedLicense.com website.
[34] MedLicense.com - Practical Advise for Physicians Who Are Involved In Telemedicine (http://www.medlicense.com/telemedicine_advice.html), MedLicense.com website.
[35] IST's Media Collection (http://www.intersurgtech.com/media.html), Interface Surgical Technologies website. Retrieved 21 August 2011.
[36] McGraw-Hill Concise Encyclopedia of Engineering. Videotelephony (http://encyclopedia2.thefreedictionary.com/Videotelephony), McGraw-Hill, 2002. Retrieved from the FreeDictionary.com website, January 9, 2010

Further reading

- W. John Blyth. "Telecommunications, Concepts, Development, and Management", Second Edition, Glencoe/McCgraw-Hill Company,1990, pp. 280–282.
- Teleneurology and requirements of the european Medical Devices Directive (MDD) (http://www.baaske.net/index.php?id=37&L=1) - Telemedical Systems and regulatory affairs for Europe, by Dipl. Ing. Armin Gärtner
- Telemedicine 101: Telemedicine Coming of Age (http://tie.telemed.org/articles/article.asp?path=telemed101&article=tmcoming_nb_tie96.xml) - Telemedicine 101: Telemedicine Coming of Age, by Nancy Brown
- What is Telemedicine? (http://www.icucare.com/PageFiles/Telemedicine.pdf) - What is Telemedicine?, by Robert Higgs (www.icucare.com)
- Critical Care 24/7 (http://www.healthmgttech.com/index.php/features/thought-leaders/critical-care-247.html) by Christina Thielst

External links

- Telemedicine and Telehealth (http://www.teladoc.com/) Teladoc.
- Telemedicine Pakistan (TelmedPak) (http://www.telmedpak.com)
- Wiki for telemedicine (ATAwiki) (http://www.ATAwiki.org)
- Agency for Healthcare Research and Quality (AHRQ) -- Telemedicine for the Medicare Population (http://www.ahrq.gov/clinic/epcsums/telemedsum.htm)
- Ontario Telemedicine Network -- Making the Connection for Health (http://www.otn.ca)
- American Telemedicine Association (http://www.americantelemed.org)
- Telemedicine Information Exchange (http://tie.telemed.org)
- Canadian Society of Telehealth (http://www.cst-sct.org)
- TELESYNERGY - Telemedicine at the National Institutes of Health (http://telesynergy.nih.gov)
- Telemedicine History (http://www.depts.ttu.edu/communications/vistas/archive/02-summer/stories/miracle-of-telemedicine.php)
- National Rural Health Association (http://www.nrharural.org)
- International Society for Telemedicine & eHealth (ISfTeH) (http://www.isft.net)

- American Psychiatric Asscoiation (http://www.psych.org/Departments/HSF/UnderservedClearinghouse/Linkeddocuments/telepsychiatry.aspx)

Telehealth

Telehealth is the delivery of health-related services and information via telecommunications technologies. Telehealth could be as simple as two health professionals discussing a case over the telephone or as sophisticated as doing robotic surgery between facilities at different ends of the globe.

Telehealth is an expansion of telemedicine, and unlike telemedicine (which more narrowly focuses on the curative aspect) it encompasses preventive, promotive *and* curative aspects. Originally used to describe administrative or educational functions related to telemedicine, today telehealth stresses a myriad of technology solutions. For example, physicians use email to communicate with patients, order drug prescriptions and provide other health services.

Clinical uses of telehealth technologies

- Transmission of medical images for diagnosis (often referred to as store and forward telehealth)
- Groups or individuals exchanging health services or education live via videoconference (real-time telehealth)
- Transmission of medical data for diagnosis or disease management (sometimes referred to as remote monitoring)
- Advice on prevention of diseases and promotion of good health by patient monitoring and followup.
- Health advice by telephone in emergent cases (referred to as teletriage)

Nonclinical uses of telehealth technologies

- Distance education including continuing medical education, grand rounds, and patient education
- administrative uses including meetings among telehealth networks, supervision, and presentations
- research on telehealth
- online information and health data management
- healthcare system integration
- asset identification, listing, and patient to asset matching, and movement
- overall healthcare system management
- patient movement and remote admission

Telehealth modes

Store-and-forward telehealth

In store-and-forward telehealth, digital images, video, audio, observations of daily living (ODLs),[1] and clinical data are captured and "stored" on the client computer or mobile device; then at a convenient time they are transmitted securely ("forwarded") to a clinic at another location where they are studied by relevant specialists. The opinion of the specialist is then transmitted back. Based on the requirements of the participating healthcare entities, this roundtrip could take between 1 minute to 48 hours. In the simplest form of telehealth application, basic vital signs like blood pressure, weight, pulse oximeter, and blood sugar values are monitored and trended for long term chronic care. In many specialties, such as dermatology, radiology and pathology, an immediate response is not critical, making these specialties conducive to store-and-forward technologies. Automated screening and diagnostic tele-audiology is fast becoming another specialty conducive to store-and-forward audiology.

Real-time telehealth

In real-time telehealth, a telecommunications link allows instantaneous interaction. Videoconferencing equipment is one of the most common forms of synchronous telemedicine. Peripheral devices can also be attached to computers or the video-conferencing equipment which can aid in an interactive examination. With the availability of better and cheaper communication channels, direct two-way audio and video streaming between centers through computers is leading to lower costs.

Examples of real-time clinical telehealth include:

- Tele-audiology
- Telecardiology
- Teledentistry
- Telemental Health -- the use of videoconferencing technology to connect a psychiatrist with a mental health client
- Teleneurology
- Telenursing
- Teleradiology
- Telerehabilitation

In an effort to enhance the real-time telehealth experience, Google Health, a personal health information centralization service, recently began establishing relationships with telehealth providers that will allow their users to sync the data shared during telehealth consultations with their online health records. To date, partnerships have been formed with the following companies: MDLiveCare and Hello Health.[2]

In the UK Stoke on Trent Primary Care Trust together with mediaburst and the West Midlands Strategic Health Authority have sponsored the development of a low cost Simple Telehealth [3] system "Florence [4]" which primarily operates using text messaging (SMS) and a web application.

Remote patient monitoring

In remote monitoring, sensors are used to capture and transmit physiological data. For example, a tele-EEG device monitors the electrical activity of a patients brain and then transmits that data to a specialist. This could be done in either real time or the data could be stored and then forwarded.

Examples of remote monitoring include:

- Home-based nocturnal dialysis [5]
- Cardiac and multi-parameter monitoring of remote ICUs
- Home telehealth
- Disease management

Benefits of telehealth

Telehealth adds a new paradigm in healthcare, where the patient is monitored between physician office visits. This has been shown to significantly reduce hospitalizations and visits to the Emergency Room, while improving patient's quality of life. Telehealth also benefits patients where traditional delivery of health services are affected by distance and lack of local specialist clinicians to deliver services.

The rate of adoption of telehealth services in any jurisdiction is frequently influenced by factors such as the adequacy and cost of existing conventional health services in meeting patient needs; the policies of governments and/or insurers with respect to coverage and payment for telehealth services; and medical licensing requirements that may inhibit or deter the provision of telehealth second opinions or primary consultations by physicians.

There may also be some significant carbon reductions for the NHS to be gained from developing Telehealth and therefore reducing the need to travel (often, in the case of patients, by car) as well as encouraging healthy, sustainable behaviour through monitoring and improved communications and reducing the requirements to expand sites to meet increases in Healthcare demands.

The state of the market

Projections for the growth of the telehealth market are optimistic, and much of this optimism is predicated upon the increasing demand for remote medical care. According to a recent survey, nearly three-quarters of U.S. consumers say they would use telehealth.[6] At present, several major companies are scrambling to establish a foothold in a market that, according to market-research firm Datamonitor, is expected to grow to more than $6 billion by 2012 from 900 million in 2007.[7]

See also

- Ontario Telemedicine Network
- List of video telecommunication services and product brands
- Tele-epidemiology
- Telemedicine
- eHealth
- mHealth
- American Telemedicine Association
- National Rural Health Association
- Connected Health
- Remote therapy

References

[1] Health in Everyday Living (http://www.projecthealthdesign.org/media/file/E-primer_3.pdf) Robert Wood Johnson Foundation primer.

[2] "Fall update on Google Health" (http://googleblog.blogspot.com/2009/10/fall-update-on-google-health.html). . Retrieved 2009-10-07.

[3] http://www.stoke.nhs.uk/simple

[4] http://www.getflorence.co.uk/

[5] Andreas Pierratos, MD. Nocturnal hemodialysis: dialysis for the new millennium (http://www.cmaj.ca/cgi/content/full/161/9/1137) Canadian Medical Association Journal, November 2, 1999; 161 (9), 2 November 1966.

[6] "Survey: Consumers Keen on Telemedicine" (http://www.healthdatamanagement.com/news/telemedicine-38701-1.html). . Retrieved 2010-04-26.

[7] "Homecare telehealth expected to grow despite current barriers to adoption" (http://it.tmcnet.com/news/2007/08/30/2897900.htm). . Retrieved 2010-04-26.

Further reading

- Telemedicine,Telehealth, and the Consumer (http://tie.telemed.org/articles/article.asp?path=consumer&article=tmcoming_nb_tie96.xml) Online introduction and primer to telehealth and telemedicine from the Telemedicine Information Exchange
- Norris, A. C. (2002). *Essentials of Telemedicine and Telecare*. West Sussex, England; New York: John Wiley & Sons, Ltd. ISBN 0-471-53151-0.
- Maheu, Marlene M.; Whitten, Pamela; & Allen, Ace (2001). *E-Health, Telehealth, and Telemedicine: A Guide to Start-up and Success*. San Francisco: Jossey Bass. ISBN 0-7879-4420-3.
- Olmeda, Christopher J. (2000). Information Technology in Systems of Care. Delfin Press. ISBN 978-0-9821442-0-6
- Telehealth Technical Assistance Manual (http://www.nrharural.org/pubs/pdf/Telehealth.pdf) - A document to assist in the planning of telehealth and telemedicine projects for rural community and migrant health centers and other health care organizations. By Samuel G. Burgess, Ph.D. October 2006

- Teleneurology and requirements of the european Medical Devices Directive (MDD) (http://www.baaske.net/index.php?id=37&L=1) - Telemedical Systems and regulatory affairs for Europe, by Dipl. Ing. Armin Gärtner

External links

- Telehealth connectivity between Patients, Nurse Practitioners, General Practitioners, Specialists and Allied Health Professionals (http://www.telehealthnetworks.com.au/).Telehealth Networks.
- Telehealth for Patients, Providers, Health Plans, Employers (http://www.americanwell.com/). American Well.
- Telemedicine and Telehealth (http://www.teladoc.com/). Teladoc.
- Post discharge follow-up calls (http://www.telenursefirst.com/). TeleNurse First.
- Center for Telehealth and Technology (http://t2health.org/) DOD Defense Centers of Excellence
- Telehealth wiki (http://www.ATAwiki.org)
- Telemental Health Guide (http://www.tmhguide.org)
- HealthLink BC (http://www.HealthLinkBC.ca)
- Telehealth Ontario (http://www.health.gov.on.ca/english/public/program/telehealth/telehealth_mn.html)
- Ontario Telemedicine Network -- Making the Connection for Health (http://www.otn.ca)
- Tasmanian government (http://www.dhhs.tas.gov.au/service_information/services_files/telecare)
- GP2U Telehealth Australia (http://gp2u.com.au/)
- NHS Direct (http://www.nhsdirect.nhs.uk/), the UK National Health Service information service
- NHS Stoke on Trent (http://www.stoke.nhs.uk/simple) Simple Telehealth Project
- International Society for Telemedicine & eHealth (http://www.isft.net/)
- Med-e-Tel - The International Educational and Networking Forum for eHealth, Telemedicine and Health ICT (http://www.medetel.lu/)
- Community for Teledermatology (http://telederm.org)
- Scottish Centre for Telehealth (http://www.sct.scot.nhs.uk)
- British Columbia Alliance on Telehealth Policy and Research (http://www.bcatpr.ca)
- UCLA Wireless Health Institute (http://www.wirelesshealth.ucla.edu)
- Fit for the Future, Scenarios for low-carbon healthcare in 2030 (http://www.forumforthefuture.org/files/Fit_for_the_Future_NHS_Sept09.pdf)
- Lifesize Case Study on Telehealth (http://www.lifesize.com/Industry_Solutions/Case_Studies/Case-Study_Village-Church.aspx)

United States oriented

- Office for the Advancement of Telehealth (http://telehealth.hrsa.gov/index.htm) (established by the Health Resources and Services Administration)
- U.S. Department of Veterans Affairs Care Coordination/Telehealth Program (http://www.carecoordination.va.gov)
- American Telemedicine Association (http://www.americantelemed.org)
- National Rural Health Association (http://www.NRHArural.org/)
- National Center for Telehealth & Technology (http://www.t2health.org)
- Center for Telehealth & E-Health Law (http://www.telehealthlawcenter.org)
- Telemedicine Information Exchange (http://tie.telemed.org/)
- University of New Mexico Telehealth (http://hsc.unm.edu/som/telehealth/)
- University of Florida Center for Telehealth (http://telehealth.phhp.ufl.edu/)

ECare_(software)

eCare is a web-based remote support application developed by Motorola and designed to be used by help desks, consultants, and customer service organizations to assist and support their clients across the Internet. It can integrate into existing customer relationship management (CRM) systems, as well as operate on its own. eCare's main functionality includes chat, file transfer, remote control, remote diagnostics, and scripting.

External links

- eCare product information page at Motorola [1]

References

[1] http://www.netopia.com/software/products/ecare/

Assistive_technology

Assistive technology or **adaptive technology** (AT) is an umbrella term that includes assistive, adaptive, and rehabilitative devices for people with disabilities and also includes the process used in selecting, locating, and using them. AT promotes greater independence by enabling people to perform tasks that they were formerly unable to accomplish, or had great difficulty accomplishing, by providing enhancements to, or changing methods of interacting with, the technology needed to accomplish such tasks.

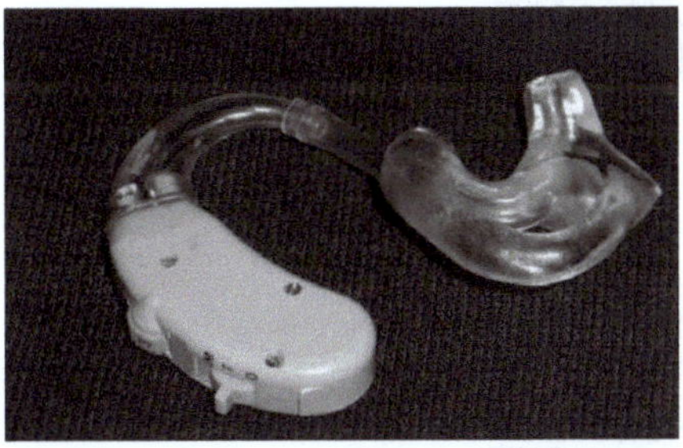

Hearing aid

Likewise, disability advocates point out that technology is often created without regard to people with disabilities, creating unnecessary barriers to hundreds of millions of people. Even the makers of AT technologies will often still argue that universal design is preferable to the need for AT and that universal design projects and concepts should be continuously expanded.

Overview

Assistive Technology is a generic term for devices and modifications that help overcome or remove a disability. The first recorded example of the use of a prosthesis dates to at least 1800 BC.[1] and the modern, lightweight, steel, collapsible wheelchair was created by Harry Jennings and his disabled friend Herbert Everest, in 1933[2] .

Examples of Assistive technology in architecture include the curb cut is a related structural innovation. Other examples are standing frames, text telephones, accessible keyboards, large print, Braille, & speech recognition computer software. People with disabilities often develop personal or community adaptations, such as strategies to suppress tics in public (for example in Tourette's syndrome), or sign language in deaf communities. Assistive technology or interventions are sometimes controversial or rejected, for example in the controversy over cochlear implants for children.

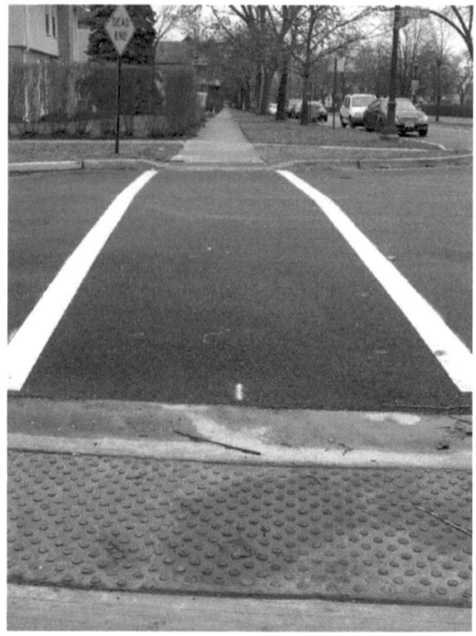

Universally Accessible Street Cross at Evanston, Illinois

Universally accessible technology yields great rewards to the typical user as well; good accessible design *is* universal design. One example is the "curb cuts" (or dropped curbs) in the sidewalk at street crossings. While these curb cuts enable pedestrians with mobility impairments to cross the street, they also aid parents with carriages and strollers, shoppers with carts, and travelers and workers with pull-type bags.

People with learning disabilities like dyslexia or dysgraphia can find text-to-speech (TTS) software useful for reading and spelling programs useful when writing texts.

Computers, with their hardware extensibility, editing, spellchecking and speech synthesis software are becoming the cornerstone of assistive technologies, improving quality of life for those with learning disabilities and visual impairments. Spell assist programs and voice-recognition facilities are also bringing the text reading and writing experience to the wider public.

Toys that have been adapted to be used by children with disabilities might have advantages for non-disabled children as well. The Lekotek movement assists parents by lending assistive technology toys and expertise to families.

In the US many health professionals may be certified by RESNA to serve assistive technology needs: occupational therapists, physical therapists, speech language pathologists/audiologists, orthotists and prosthetists, educators, and rehabilitation and health professionals.

Assistive technology products

Personal Emergency Response Systems

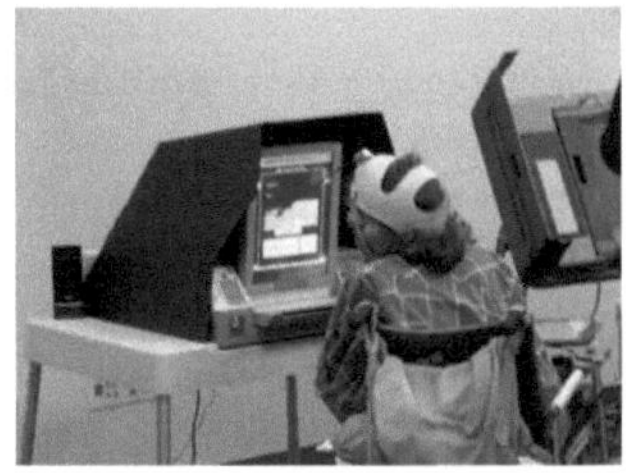

This voter with a manual dexterity disability is making choices on a touchscreen with a head dauber.

Personal Emergency Response Systems (PERS), or Telecare (UK term), are a particular sort of assistive technology that use electronic sensors connected to an alarm system to help caregivers manage risk and help vulnerable people stay independent at home longer. An example would be the systems being put in place for senior people such as fall detectors, thermometers (for hypothermia risk), flooding and unlit gas sensors (for people with mild dementia). Notably, these alerts can be customized to the particular person's risks. When the alert is triggered, a message is sent to a caregiver or contact center who can respond appropriately.

Technology similar to PERS can also be used to act within a person's home rather than just to respond to a detected crisis. Using one of the examples above, gas sensors for people with dementia can be used to trigger a device that turns off the gas and tells someone what has happened.

Designing for people with dementia is a good example of how the design of the interface of a piece of AT is critical to its usefulness. People with dementia or any other identified user group must be involved in the design process to make sure that the design is accessible and usable. In the example above, a voice message could be used to remind the person with dementia to turn off the gas himself, but whose voice should be used, and what should the message say? Questions like these must be answered through user consultation, involvement and evaluation.

Accessible Input devices for Computers

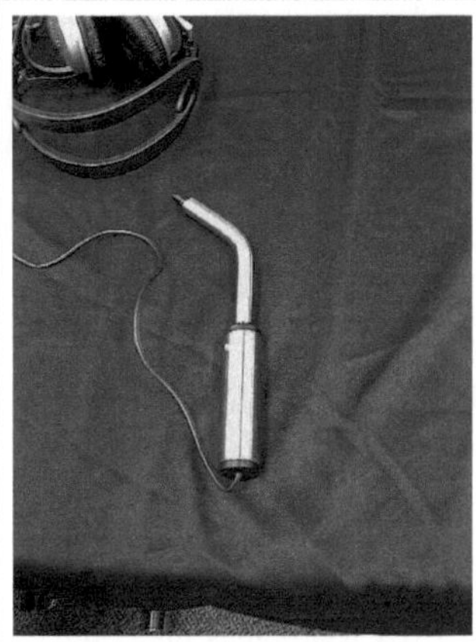

This is a sip-and-puff device which allows a person with substantial disability to make selections and navigate computerized interfaces by controlling inhalations and exhalations.

Sitting at a desk with a QWERTY keyboard and a mouse remains the dominant way of interacting with a personal computer. Some Assistive Technology reduces the strain of this way of work through ergonomic accessories with height-adjustable furniture, footrests, wrist rests, and arm supports to ensure correct posture. Key guards fit over the keyboard to help prevent unintentional key presses.

Alternatively, Assistive Technology may attempt to improve the ergonomics of the devices themselves:

- Ergonomic keyboards reduce the discomfort and strain of typing.
- Chorded keyboards have a handful of keys (one per digit per hand) to type by 'chords' which produce different letters and keys.
- Expanded keyboards with larger, more widely spaced keys.
- Compact and miniature keyboards.
- Dvorak and other alternative layouts may offer more ergonomic layouts of the keys.[3] [4] There are also variants of Dvorak in which the most common keys are located at either the left or right side of the keyboard.

Input devices may be modified to make them easier to see and understand:

- Keyboards with lowercase keys
- Keyboards with big keys.

- Keyboards with less and big keys, or multifunctional keys, such us the special keyboard PiTech, with only five big rounded keys, which is used with a special software for writing[5]
- Large print keyboard with high contrast colors (such as white on black, black on white, and black on ivory).
- Large print adhesive keyboard stickers in high contrast colors (such as white on black, black on white, and black on yellow).
- Embossed locator dots help find the 'home' keys, F and J, on the keyboard.
- Scroll wheels on mice remove the need to locate the scrolling interface on the computer screen.
- Footmouse — Foot-operated mouse.

More ambitiously, and quite crucially when keyboard or mouse prove unusable, AT can also replace the keyboard and mouse with alternative devices such as the LOMAK keyboard, trackballs, joysticks, graphics tablets, touchpads, touch screens, foot mice, a microphone with speech recognition software, sip-and-puff input, switch access, and vision-based input devices, such as eye trackers which allow the user to control the mouse with their eyes.

Accessibility Software

In human-computer interaction, computer accessibility (also known as Accessible computing) refers to the accessibility of a computer system to all people, regardless of disability or severity of impairment. Examples include Web accessibility a set of guidelines [6] and two accessible[7] web portals designed for people developing reading skills are peepo.com [8] — try typing a letter with your keyboard for more — and peepo.co.uk [9] with enhanced graphics, unique style controls and improved interactivity (requires an SVG supported browser).

Durable Medical Equipment (DME)

- Seating products that assist people to sit comfortably and safely (seating systems, cushions, therapeutic seats).
- Standing products to support people with disabilities in the standing position while maintaining/improving their health (standing frame, standing wheelchair, active stander).
- Walking products to aid people with disabilities who are able to walk or stand with assistance (canes, crutches, walkers, gait trainers).
- Advanced technology walking products to aid people with disabilities, such as paraplegia or cerebral palsy, who would not at all able to walk or stand (exoskeletons).
- Wheeled mobility products that enable people with reduced mobility to move freely indoors and outdoors (wheelchairs/scooters)
- Vehicles modified with Height adjustable suspension, to allow wheelchair entry to the vehicle
- Robot-aided rehabilitation is a sensory-motor rehabilitation technique based on the use of robots and mechatronic devices

Mobility impairment

- Crutches, including assistive canes
- Walkers
- Wheelchairs

Assistive technology for visual impairment

Many people with serious visual impairments live independently, using a wide range of tools and techniques. Examples of assistive technology for visually impairment is include the Canadian currency tactile feature, which a system of raised dots in one corner, based on Braille cells but not standard Braille.[10] . For general computer use access technology such as screen readers, screen magnifiers and refreshable Braille displays has been widely taken up.

Hardware

- White canes
- Large monitors can be used with increased DPI for ease of electronic text reading.
- E-book readers, such as the Amazon Kindle and tablet computers, such as the iPad, which offer text-to-speech and adjustable font size features.
- Adjustable task lamp, using a fluorescent bulb, shines directly onto the paper and can be adjusted to suit.
- Bank note reader
- Copyholder holds printed material in near vertical position for easier reading and can be adjusted to suit.
- Closed circuit television (CCTV) or video magnifiers. Printed materials and objects are placed under a camera and the magnified image is displayed onto a screen.
- Modified cassette recorder. To record a lecture, own thoughts, ideas, notes etc.
- Desktop compact cassette dictation system. To allow audio cassette playback with the aid of a foot pedal.
- Fusers produce tactile materials, for example diagrams and maps, by applying heat to special swell paper.
- Scanner. A device used in conjunction with OCR software. The printed document is scanned and converted into electronic text, which can then be displayed on screen as recognizable text.
- Standalone reading aids integrate a scanner, optical character recognition (OCR) software, and speech software in a single machine. These function together without a separate PC.[11]
- Refreshable Braille display. An electronic tactile device which is placed below the computer keyboard. A line of cells which correspond to Braille text move up and down to represent a line of text on the computer screen.
- Electronic Notetaker. A portable computer with a Braille or QWERTY keyboard and synthetic speech. Some models have an integrated Braille display.
- Braille embosser. Embosses Braille output from a computer by punching dots onto paper. It connects to a computer in the same way as a text printer.
- Perkins Brailler. To manually emboss Grade 1 or 2 Braille.
- Mountbatten Brailler. An electric braille writing machine.
- Eye Tracking. and Head Tracking Devices

Software

- Customization of graphical user interfaces to alter the colors and size of desktops, short-cut icons, menu bars and scroll bars.
- Screen magnifiers
- Screen readers
- Self-voicing applications
- Optical character recognition. Converts the printed word into text, via a scanner.
- Braille translation. Converts the printed word into Braille, which can then be embossed via a Braille embosser.
- Text-to-speech and Speech-to-text
- Spell checkers and Grammar checkers
- Real-time text for the deaf.

Augmentative and Alternative Communication (AAC)

Augmentative and alternative communication (AAC) is an umbrella term that encompasses methods of communication for those with impairments or restrictions on the production or comprehension of spoken or written language.[12] AAC systems are extremely diverse and depend on the capabilities of the user. They may be as basic as pictures on a board that the are used to request food, drink, or other care; or they can be advanced speech generating devices, based on speech synthesis, that are capable of storing hundreds of phrases and words.[13]

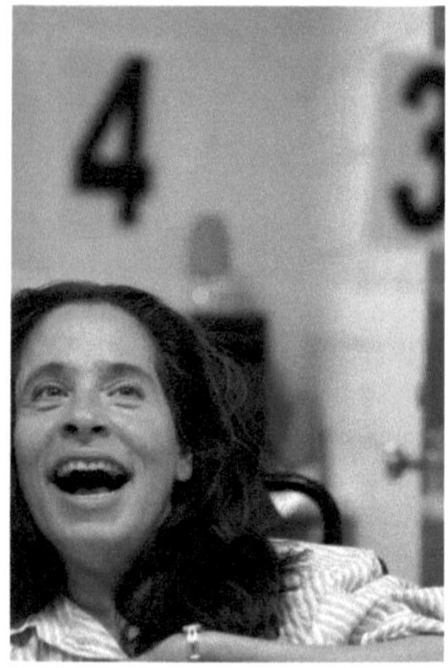

An AAC user uses number coding on an eye gaze communication board

Modern use of AAC began in the 1950s with systems for users who had lost the use of speech following surgical procedures.[14] During the 1960s the use of manual sign language grew greatly, but it was not until the 1980s that AAC began to emerge as an area in its own right.[14] AAC is now used for a wide variety of speech impairments. Studies show that AAC use does not impede the development of speech, and may even result in a modest increase in speech production.[15]

A great diversity of diagnoses, including cerebral palsy, intellectual impairment, autism, and many others, cover varying degrees of communication impairment. AAC interventions are highly individualized, taking into account specific abilities of language comprehension, social-relational characteristics, learning strengths and weaknesses, and developmental patterns for specific types of intellectual disabilities.[16] AAC can be used to aid both spoken and written language, and can supplement or replace speech and writing as necessary. AAC can be a permanent addition to a person's communication or a temporary aid.[12] The systems used in AAC include gestures, hand signals, photographs, pictures, line drawings, words and letters,[17] which can be used alone or in combination to communicate.[18]

Aided AAC makes great use of symbols, particularly for non-literate users,[17] as well as a large variety of input methods. The specific access method will depend on the skills and abilities of the user. Body parts, pointers, adapted mice, joysticks, or eye tracking[19] could be used, whereas switch access scanning is often used for indirect selection.[20] In many cases, rate enhancements methods may be used to speed up the generation of messages.[17] Clearly, an evaluation of a user's abilities and requirements is necessary to match a user with the most appropriate AAC method, input approach, and vocabulary. This evaluation requires the input of family, particularly for early intervention. Respecting ethnicity and family beliefs are key to a family-centered and ethnically competent approach.[21] Adult AAC users generally have satisfying relationships with family and friends and engage in pleasurable and interesting life activities.

Deafness and hearing loss

- Audiometer
- Fire alarm paging system
- Loop system (portable and fixed)
- Radio aids
- Telecommunications device for the deaf
- Teletext
- Video cassette recorders that can read and record subtitles (Closed Captioning).
- Vibrating fire alarm placed under pillow when asleep.
- Door bell lighting system.

Others

- Wakamaru provides companionship, reminds users to take medicine and calls for help if something is wrong.
- Telephone Reassurance: community based program that calls seniors at home ensuring their well-being.[22]
- Cosmobot is part of a play therapy system designed to motivate children to participate in therapy.
- General User Interface for Disorders of Execution (GUIDE) is an interactive verbal prompting system that talks people with cognitive impairment through daily routine tasks.[23]

Claims Since children with autism process visual information easier than auditory information, when utilizing assistive technology claims that any time we use these devices with these children, we're giving them information through their strongest processing area (visual). Therefore various types of technology from "low" tech to "high" tech, should be incorporated into every aspect of daily living in order to improve the functional capabilities of children with autism.

Benefits Regarding comprehension skills, increasing comprehension of tasks/activities/situations is essential in addressing skill areas such as organization, attending, self help, following directions, following rules and modifying behavior. As a result, the child becomes more independent. The following "low" tech visual support strategies can be created and used to benefit and assist the child in increasing his comprehension skills and thus decreasing the occurrence of challenging behaviors.

Consistent daily use of an individualized visual schedule will increase a child's organization skills and independent functioning throughout all aspects of his life and will ease transition through adulthood. There are numerous ways to present visual schedules for example an object schedule, 3-ring binder schedule, clipboard schedule, manila file folder schedules, and dry erase board schedules are all beneficial to increase a child's organization skills and independent functioning.

The use of a weekly/monthly calendar at both home and school can provide the child with important information regarding up-coming events/activities, rather than relying on auditory information. When the child asks when a particular event will occur, he can easily be referred to the visual calendar. Use of a visual calendar can also be helpful in assisting the child to understand when regularly scheduled events may not occur.

Outcomes In a pilot study, Researchers Lacava, Golan, Baron-Cohen, and Myles explored the use of assistive technology to teach emotion recognition to eight children with Autism and the results indicated that after intervention, participants improved on face and voice emotional recognition for basic and complex emotions that were in the software. As well as for complex voice emotional recognition for emotions not included in Mind Reading.

See also

- Braille technology
- Cognitive orthotics
- Design for All (in ICT)
- Matching Person & Technology Model
- OATS: Open Source Assistive Technology Software
- Occupational Therapy
- Web accessibility

Notes

[1] Disability Social History Project (http://www.disabilityhistory.org/timeline_new.html)
[2] Everest, Herbert A., Jennings, Harry C., "Folding wheel chair", US Patent 2095411, 1937
[3] Chubon, R.A., Hester, M.R. (1988). "An enhanced standard computer keyboard system for single-finger and typing-stick typing". *Journal of Rehabilitation Research and Development* **25** (4): 17–24. PMID 2973523.
[4] Anson, D., George, S., Galup, R., Shea, B., Vetter, R. (2001). "Efficiency of the Chubon versus the QWERTY keyboard". *Assistive-Technology* **13** (1): 40–5. doi:10.1080/10400435.2001.10132032. PMID 12212435.
[5] PiTech (http://www.pitech.com.ar)
[6] http://www.learningdisabilities.org.uk/page.cfm?pagecode=ISSIWD
[7] http://www.learningdisabilities.org.uk/page.cfm?pagecode=ISSIWDAS
[8] http://www.peepo.com
[9] http://www.peepo.co.uk
[10] Accessibility features - Bank Notes - Bank of Canada (http://www.bankofcanada.ca/en/banknotes/accessibility.html)
[11] "What is an electronic reading aid?" (http://www.rnib.org.uk/livingwithsightloss/Documents/What is an electronic reading aid.doc). Royal National Institute of Blind People (http://www.rnib.org.uk/). 2009-12-01. . Retrieved 2010-02-23.
[12] ASHA (2005).
[13] Gilliam & Marquardt, pp. 356–359.
[14] Glennen & DeCoste.
[15] Schlosser & Wendt.
[16] Beukelman & Mirenda.
[17] Mirenda.
[18] Beukelman & Mirenda, pp. 246-249.
[19] Mathy
[20] Jans & Clark.
[21] Perette et al. (2000).
[22] assistivetech.net: Telephone Reassurance (http://atwiki.assistivetech.net/index.php/Telephone_Reassurance). Accessed 2009-08-06.
[23] Brian O'Neill, Kate Moran, Alex Gillespie (2010). "Scaffolding rehabilitation behaviour using a voice mediated assistive technology for cognition" (http://www.psychology.stir.ac.uk/staff/agillespie/documents/ONeillMoranGillespie_Scaffoldingrehabilitationbehaviour.pdf). *Neuropsychological Rehabilitation* **18**: 1–19. .

References

- American Speech-Language-Hearing Association. (2005). "Roles and Responsibilities of Speech-Language Pathologists With Respect to Augmentative and Alternative Communication: Position Statement" (http://www.asha.org/docs/html/PS2005-00113.html). Retrieved 2009-01-23.
- Gillam, Ronald Bradley; Marquardt, Thomas P.; Martin, Frederick N. (2000). *Communication sciences and disorders: from science to clinical practice*. Jones & Bartlett Learning. ISBN 9780769300405.
- DeCoste, Denise C. (1997). "Chapter 10: Introduction to Augmentative and Alternative Communication Systems". In Glennen, Sharon; DeCoste, Denise C.. *Handbook Of Augmentative And Alternative Communication*. San Diego, CA: Singular Publishing Group. ISBN 1-56593-684-1.
- Schlosser, R. W.; Wendt, O. (2008). "Effects of augmentative and alternative communication intervention on speech production in children with autism: a systematic review". *American Journal of Speech-Language Pathology* **17** (3): 212–230. doi:10.1044/1058-0360(2008/021). PMID 18663107.

- Beukelman, David R.; Mirenda, Pat (2005). *Augmentative & alternative communication: supporting children & adults with complex communication needs* (3rd ed.). Paul H. Brookes Publishing Company. ISBN 9781557666840.
- Mirenda, P. (2003). "Toward Functional Augmentative and Alternative Communication for Students With Autism: Manual Signs, Graphic Symbols, and Voice Output Communication Aids". *Language, Speech, & Hearing Services in Schools* **34** (3): 203–216. doi:10.1044/0161-1461(2003/017).
- Mathy; Yorkston, K.; Guttman (2000). "Augmentative Communication for Individuals with Amyotrophic Lateral Sclerosis". In Beukelman, D.; Yorkston, K.; Reichle, J.. *Augmentative and Alternative Communication Disorders for Adults with Acquired Neurologic Disorders*. Baltimore: P. H. Brookes Pub.. ISBN 978-1557664730.
- Jans, Deborah; Clark, Sue (1998). "Chapter 6: High Technology Aids to Communication" (http://www.callscotland.org.uk/Resources/Books/Augmentative-Communication-in-Practice/). In Wilson, Allan. *Augmentative Communication in Practice: An Introduction*. University of Edinburgh. ISBN 978-1898042150.
- Parette, H. P.; Brotherson, M. J; Huer, M. B. (2000). "Giving families a voice in augmentative and alternative communication decision-making" (http://psycnet.apa.org/psycinfo/2001-17960-006). *Education and Training in Mental Retardation and Developmental Disabilities* **35**: 177–190.

Further Reading

- Behrmann, M., Schaff, J. (2001). "Assisting educators with assistive technology: Enabling children to achieve independence in living and learning". *Children and Families* **42** (3): 24–8.
- Bishop, J. (2003). "The Internet for educating individuals with social impairments" (http://www.jonathanbishop.com/publications/display.aspx?Item=9). *Journal of Computer Assisted Learning* **19** (4): 546–556. doi:10.1046/j.0266-4909.2003.00057.x.
- Cain, S. (2001). *Accessing Technology — Using technology to support the learning and employment opportunities for visually impaired users*. Royal National Institute for the Blind. ISBN 1-85878-517-0.
- Cook, A., Hussey, S. (2002). *Assistive Technologies — Principles and Practice* (2nd ed.). Mosby. ISBN 0-323-00643-4.
- Edwards, A. D. N., ed (1995). *Extra-Ordinary Human-Computer Interaction: Interfaces for Users with Disabilities*. Cambridge Series on Human-Computer Interaction. New York: Cambridge University Press. ISBN 0521434130. (Also available as part of the CD-rom, Overcoming Barriers: Theory and Practice in Disability, Cambridge University Press, 1999).
- Franklin, K.S. (1991). "Supported employment and assistive technology-A powerful partnership". In S.L. Griffin, W.G. Revell. *Rehabilitation counselor desktop guide to supported employment*. Richmond, VA: Virginia Commonwealth University Rehabilitation Research and Training Center on Supported Employment.
- Van der Heijden, D. (2005). How Does Alternative Access to Computers Work? (http://www.axistive.com/how-does-alternative-access-to-computers-work.html). Jun 26, 2007.
- Lahm, E., & Morrissette, S. (1994, April). Zap 'em with assistive technology. Paper presented at the annual meeting of The Council for Exceptional Children, Denver, CO.
- Lee, C. (1999). *Learning disabilities and assistive technologies; an emerging way to touch the future*. Amherst, MA: McGowan Publications.
- McKeown, S. (2000). *Unlocking Potential — How ICT can support children with special needs*. The Questions Publishing Company Ltd. ISBN 1-84190-041-9.
- Nisbet, P., Poon, P. (1998) (Free Download). *Special Access Technology* (http://callcentre.education.ed.ac.uk/About_CALL/Publications_CAA/Books_CAB/SAT_CAC/sat_cac.html). The CALL Centre, University of Edinburgh. ISBN 1-898042-11-X.
- Nisbet, P., Spooner, R., Arthur, E., Whittaker P. (1999) (Free Download). *Supportive Writing Technology* (http://callcentre.education.ed.ac.uk/About_CALL/Publications_CAA/Books_CAB/Supp_Writing_CAC/supp_writing_cac.html). The CALL Centre, University of Edinburgh. ISBN 1-898042-13-6.

- Rose, D., Meyer, A. (2000). "Universal design for individual differences". *Educational Leadership* **58** (3): 39–43.
- Orpwood RD (Jan-Feb 1990). "Design methodology for aids for the disabled". *J Med Eng Technol* **14** (1): 2–10. doi:10.3109/03091909009028756. PMID 2342081.
- Scherer, M. J. (2005). *Living in the State of Stuck: How Assistive Technology Impacts the Lives of People with Disabilities* (4th ed.). Cambridge, MA: Brookline Books. ISBN 1-571-29098-2.
- Scherer, M. J. (2004). *Connecting to Learn: Educational and Assistive Technology for People with Disabilities.* Washington, DC: American Psychological Association (APA) Books. ISBN 1-557-98982-6.
- Scherer, M. J., ed (2002). *Assistive Technology: Matching Device and Consumer for Successful Rehabilitation.* Washington, DC: APA Books. ISBN 1-557-98840-4.
- Swann, J. I. (2007). *Promoting independence and activity in older people.* Quay Books. ISBN 9781856423342.
- Adlam, T., *et al.* (2004). "The installation and support of internationally distributed equipment for people with dementia" (http://ieeexplore.ieee.org/iel5/4233/29401/01331402.pdf) (PDF). *IEEE Transactions on Information Technology in Biomedicine* **8** (3): 253–7. doi:10.1109/TITB.2004.834393. PMID 15484430.
- Poulson, David; Martin Ashby; Simon Richardson (eds.) (1996). *userfit. A practical handbook on user-centred design for Assistive Technology.* TIDE USER consortium.

Wandering_(dementia)

Wandering, in persons with dementia, is a common behavior that can cause great risk for the person, and is often the major priority (and concern) for caregivers. It is estimated to be the most common form disruption from people with dementia within institutions.[1] Although it occurs in several types of dementia, wandering is especially common in persons with Alzheimer's disease (AD). This can be due to forgetfulness, and also to a frequent need for stimulation.

Elopement

Unattended wandering that goes out of bounds, a behavior known as **elopement**, is a special concern for caregivers and search and rescue responders. Wandering (especially if combined with sundowning) can result in the person's being lost out of doors at night, dressed inappropriately, and unable to take many ordinarily routine steps to ensure his or her personal safety and security. This is a situation of great urgency, and the necessity of searching at night imposes added risks on the searchers.

In some countries the social costs of elopement, already significant, are increasing rapidly.[2] A SAR mission lasting more than a few hours is likely to expend many hundreds to thousands to tens of thousands of skilled worker hours and, per mission, those involving subjects with dementia typically expend significantly more resources than others.[2]

Assessment

Assessment of a person's risk of wandering often is neglected. A review of medical records of 83 persons with dementia resident in Los Angeles, California, found that only 8% of the records included a wandering risk assessment.[3] Assessment can be performed by a social worker. In the United States the Alzheimer's Association has developed a program called "Safe Return", that includes assessment tools. An assessment tool designed for use in nursing homes is the Revised Algase Wandering Scale-Nursing Home Version (RAWS-NH); this tool may be suitable for use also in assisted living facilities.[4]

Wandering prevention

The most common form of wandering prevention is for a caregiver to remain in the company of the person likely to wander, so the caregiver can either accompany him or prevent him from wandering when the situation occurs.

Other methods used to prevent wandering, or simply to reduce the risk of wandering out of bounds, include: drugs, physical restraints, physical barriers, 24-hour real-time surveillance, and tracking devices. All of these methods have ethical issues and one, use of physical restraints, is widely considered to be inhumane.[5] Tracking devices of several kinds have been evaluated.[6] [7]

Much of the literature on wandering concerns persons resident in institutions. Studies on wandering from private residences are insufficient for comparison of prevention via drugs versus other methods.[8]

The risk of wandering can be reduced by several low-tech and minimally intrusive techniques, including: placing a visual barrier such as a curtain across a doorway.[9]

Wandering can be due to a person searching for stimulation. If a wanderer does not purposefully attempt to escape the location where they are, a minimal barrier can deter wandering behaviour. However, some wanderers will look for a familiar route from their past, while others will simply 'explore.'

Some cases of wanderers operating vehicles and driving either aimlessly or along a familiar route have been reported.

In response to wandering seniors, 25 states have adopted Silver Alert programs. Silver Alert is a program similar to AMBER Alert to notify the public of missing seniors with dementia and other cognitive disabilities.

Technology

In other efforts to help keep residents safe, mitigate liability, and protect reputations, Long Term Care and Assisted Living Facilities may use radio frequency (RFID) products to protect their residents. A resident wears a wrist, pendant, or ankle transmitter. This RFID tag can be read by receiving antenna units, which are placed usually at door or hallway locations that are deemed likely routes of egress and need monitoring. The system will then either sound an alarm or briefly lock a door [10] when a door monitor reads a transmitter worn by a resident that is at risk for wandering. This helps prevent an elopement as staff can be notified by alarms at the door, pocket pagers, and email. A caregiver will be able to quickly find the person at risk and keep them safely inside. Smaller scale versions of this technology are also used in private residences.[11]

Newer versions of this equipment have become more advanced. The newest types of systems may have the ability to: identify a RFID tag by a specific resident and forward that name to the staff; give staff a last known location of the resident; show a photo of the resident at the staff station with a mapped out door location; report the frequency, times and severity of the incidents; and finally, integrate with other access control systems, HVAC, fire alarm equipment and phone equipment.

The reason this type of system seems to be preferable is that it helps monitor those at risk for wandering and elopements while not infringing on the freedom of other residents or visitors to a facility.

References

[1] U.S. Congress, Office of Technology Assessment (1992). *Special care units for people with Alzheimer's and other dementias: Consumer education, research, regulatory, and reimbursement issues.* (http://books.google.com/?id=0SXq4vuQM6oC). Government Printing Office. ISBN 9781428928176. .

[2] "Wandering and Alzheimer's overview" (http://www.dbs-sar.com/SAR_Research/wandering.htm). dbs-sar.com. . Retrieved 2008-08-26.

[3] Cherry DL, Vickrey BG, Schwankovsky L, Heck E, Plauchm M, Yep R (August 2004). "Interventions to improve quality of care: the Kaiser Permanente-Alzheimer's Association Dementia Care Project" (http://www.ajmc.com/pubMed.cfm?pii=2656). *Am J Manag Care* **10** (8): 553–60. PMID 15352531. .

[4] Beattie ER, Song J, LaGore S (2005). "A comparison of wandering behavior in nursing homes and assisted living facilities". *Res Theory Nurs Pract* **19** (2): 181–96. PMID 16025697.

[5] Robinson L, Hutchings D, Corner L, Beyer F, Dickinson H, Vanoli A, Finch T, Hughes J, Ballard C, May C, Bond J (August 2006). "A systematic literature review of the effectiveness of non-pharmacological interventions to prevent wandering in dementia and evaluation of the ethical implications and acceptability of their use" (http://www.hta.ac.uk/execsumm/summ1026.htm). *Health Technol Assess* **10** (26): iii, ix–108. PMID 16849002. .

[6] Miskelly F (September 2005). "Electronic tracking of patients with dementia and wandering using mobile phone technology" (http://ageing.oxfordjournals.org/cgi/pmidlookup?view=long&pmid=16107453). *Age Ageing* **34** (5): 497–9. doi:10.1093/ageing/afi145. PMID 16107453. .

[7] Miskelly F (May 2004). "A novel system of electronic tagging in patients with dementia and wandering" (http://ageing.oxfordjournals.org/cgi/pmidlookup?view=long&pmid=15082438). *Age Ageing* **33** (3): 304–6. doi:10.1093/ageing/afh084. PMID 15082438. .

[8] Hermans DG, Htay UH, McShane R (2007). Htay, U Hla. ed. "Non-pharmacological interventions for wandering of people with dementia in the domestic setting". *Cochrane Database Syst Rev* (1): CD005994. doi:10.1002/14651858.CD005994.pub2. PMID 17253573.

[9] Feliciano L, Vore J, LeBlanc LA, Baker JC (2004). "Decreasing entry into a restricted area using a visual barrier". *J Appl Behav Anal* **37** (1): 107–10. doi:10.1901/jaba.2004.37-107. PMC 1284486. PMID 15154224.

[10] "Why residents wanderand what you can do about it - Feature Article - Interview" (http://findarticles.com/p/articles/mi_m3830/is_4_52/ai_100204753/pg_2/?tag=content;col1). *Nursing Homes*. 2003. .

[11] http://www.ercim.org/publication/Ercim_News/enw28/leikas.html

- PMID 15014607
- PMID 14645806
- PMID 10513031

Remote_therapy

Remote Therapy, sometimes called Telemental Health Applications[1] or Internet-based Psychotherapy,[2] is a form of psychotherapy or related psychological practice in which a trained psychotherapist meets with a client or patient via telephone, cellular phone, the internet or other electronic media in place of or in additional to conventional face-to-face psychotherapy.

Initially, it was primarily intended a substitution for conventional, face-to-face therapy in which a client or patient is required to visit a psychotherapists office. Increasingly, however, academics are studying the use of electronic media in treatment to explore the possibility of providing novel and potentially more effective therapies.

After reviewing thirteen relevant studies, the authors of a meta-analytic review of psychotherapy mediated by remote communications technology concluded that:

> Remote therapy has the potential to overcome some of the barriers to conventional psychological therapy services. Telephone-based interventions are a particularly popular research focus and as a means of therapeutic communication may confer specific advantages in terms of their widespread availability and ease of operation. However, the available evidence is limited in quantity and quality. More rigorous trials are required to confirm these preliminary estimates of effectiveness.[3]

Examples

Despite the absence of complete study, remote therapy has enjoyed growing popularity as a replacement for traditional therapy and innovative practice made possible by electronic medium. Examples include:

- The US Army has initiated a program in which soldiers in combat participate in video-based relationship counseling with their partners at home.[4]
- AbilTo LLC.[5] uses remote therapy to extend the reach of evidence-based practice and introduce innovative new practices, e.g., the team-based applications of cognitive behavioral therapy utilizing a licensed therapist and behavioral coach.
- Mayo Clinic, provides remote cognitive rehabilitation sessions to patients who have had an acquired brain injury. Using an Internet-based, secure instant messaging platform, an office-based therapist conducts the rehabilitation session with the patient, who remains in or near his or her home.[6]

See also

- Telemedicine

References

[1] David Hailey, PhD; Risto Roine, MD; Arto Ohinmaa, PhD. "The Effectiveness of Telemental Health Applications: A Review" (http://publications.cpa-apc.org/media.php?mid=694&xwm=true). The Canadian Journal of Psychiatry. . Retrieved November 2008.

[2] Gregory E Simon, Evette J Ludman. "It's Time for Disruptive Innovation in Psychotherapy" (http://www.ncbi.nlm.nih.gov/pubmed/19699995). The Lancet, Vol 374. . Retrieved August 22, 2009.

[3] Penny E Bee, Peter Bower, Karina Lovell, Simon Gilbody, David Richards, Linda Gask and Pamela Roach. "Psychotherapy mediated by remote communication technologies: a meta-analytic review" (http://www.biomedcentral.com/1471-244X/8/60). TBMC Psychiatry 2008, 8:60. . Retrieved July 22, 2008.

[4] Sgt. 1st Class Adam Shaw. "Q-West Chaplains Introduce Video Teleconference Counseling for Couples" (http://www.army.mil/-news/2009/06/15/22707-q-west-chaplains-introduce-video-teleconference-counseling-for-couples/). WWW.ARMY.MIL (The Official Homepage of The United States Army). . Retrieved June 15, 2009.

[5] "Abilto's offerings" (http://abilto.com/we-can-help/). .

[6] "At-Home, Internet-Enabled Therapy Sessions Enhance Access to Cognitive Rehabilitation for Traumatic Brain Injury Patients, Leading to High Levels of Patient and Therapist Satisfaction" (http://www.innovations.ahrq.gov/content.aspx?id=1688). .

Biotronik

Type	Privately held
Industry	Medical device manufacturer
Founded	1963
Headquarters	Berlin, Germany
Website	Biotronik [1]
References: [2] [3]	

Biotronik (Biotronik SE & Co. KG;[2] Biotronik Worldwide) is a privately-held multinational biomedical technology company headquartered in Berlin, Germany. Biotronik developed the first German cardiac pacemaker in 1963 and pioneered in the creation of remotely-monitored implanted cardiac devices. The company has marketed these telemedicine technologies in Europe since 2000, in the USA since 2001, and in over 50 other countries.

Business focus

Biotronik focuses on medical devices for vascular intervention and electrotherapy of the heart. Its products include pacemakers, implantable cardioverter-defibrillators (ICD), closed-loop stimulation devices (CLS), cardiac resynchronization therapy devices (CRS), leads, catheters, a magnesium bioresorbable stent, measurement and ablation systems for electrophysiology, vascular intervention products for treatment of stenosis and occlusion in arterial vessels, guidewires, balloon catheters, stents and stent systems for coronary and peripheral diseases, and related technologies such as the external devices used to monitor implants.[4] [3]

In January 2010, the company announced its first implantation of a "leadless" cardiac monitoring device for continuous accurate detection and recording of cardiac arrhythmias without the need for any electrodes placed in the patient's heart.[5]

Telemedicine

Biotronik offers a unique system that allows a patient's implanted device to transmit information about the condition of the patient's health, and the state of the device, directly to a secure website where a physician can observe it. The system is highly integrated with a variety of telecommunication technologies, such as landline telephone, cellular telephone, Short Messaging Service (SMS), email, or fax. Depending on the type of device and its programming, which would be determined by the medical necessity in each individual, the pacemaker or ICD could alert a physician immediately in the event of an emergency cardiac event. The physician would have access to the dataflow from the device and could assess the appropriate response.[6] [7]

In addition to providing a safety net for individuals with potentially lethal illnesses of the heart, this form of telemedicine allows periodic routine physician review to occur at a distance. Patients who have implants can be monitored as necessary, without travelling to a health care facility. The safety of this approach has been confirmed in a clinical study led by the Cleveland Clinic involving over 1,443 patients enrolled from 105 North American sites. It is the first study to test remote monitoring and rapid detection of symptomatic and asymptomatic cardiac events in a prospective, randomized trial.[8] [9] [10]

As of the end of 2009, over 230,000 systems using the Biotronik technology have been implanted in heart patients, in more than 55 countries.[5]

History

Biotronik was founded in Berlin, Germany, in 1963 by physicist Max Schaldach and electrical engineer Otto Franke, who developed the first German implantable pacemaker. The company opened its North American headquarters and production facilities in Oregon, United States, when it acquired Stimulation Technology, Inc. in the 1970s. In 1993 Biotronik developed its first ICD. In 1995 the company released a number of devices for vascular intervention such as balloon catheters and stents.[11]

Biotronik's telemetry-based accessible cardiac devices were first implanted in Europe in 2000 and in the United States in 2001.[12]

Prof. Schaldach died in the crash of an aircraft he was piloting in 2001, and was succeeded by his son, Dr. Max Schaldach, as owner of the company.[13]

Biotronik claims to be "the fastest growing medical device company globally"[14] and is expanding its global workforce of over 5,000 employees.[5]

Awards

Biotronik was nominated for the "Deutscher Zukunftspreis" an award conferred by the German Federal President for achievements in technology and innovation. This prize is considered the most important national award for scientific and technological innovations which have already proven themselves on the market.[15]

External links

- Biotronik [1]

References

[1] http://www.biotronik.com/portal/home

[2] "BIOTRONIK SE & Co. KG" (http://www.hoovers.com/company/BIOTRONIK_SE__Co_KG/yrhjtftts-1.html). *Company profiles*. Hoovers. . Retrieved 3 April 2011.

[3] "BIOTRONIK, Inc. Snapshot" (http://investing.businessweek.com/research/stocks/private/snapshot.asp?privcapId=6500053). Business Week. . Retrieved 11 January 2010.

[4] "Pharmaceutical Business Review" (http://www.pharmaceutical-business-review.com/companies/biotronik_gmbh_co_kg/). . Retrieved 11 January 2010.

[5] "BIOTRONIK: Unique Leadless Cardiac Monitoring Device Implanted" (http://www.devicespace.com/news_story.aspx?StoryID=166882&full=1). 6 January 2010. . Retrieved 11 January 2010.

[6] "Unique Leadless Cardiac Monitoring Device Implanted" (http://www.streetinsider.com/Press+Releases/Unique+Leadless+Cardiac+Monitoring+Device+Implanted/5224337.html). January 6, 2010. . Retrieved 11 January 2010.

[7] "BIOTRONIK launches its new, unified platform pacemaker series in Europe" (http://www.news-medical.net/news/20091027/BIOTRONIK-launches-its-new-unified-platform-pacemaker-series-in-Europe.aspx). THE MEDICAL NEWS from News-Medical.Net. 27 October 2009. . Retrieved 11 January 2010.

[8] Varma, N; et al.. *Evaluation of efficacy and safety of remote monitoring for ICD follow-up: the TRUST trial* (http://circ.ahajournals.org/cgi/reprint/118/22/2309). **2008**. Circulation: American Heart Association. pp. 2309–2317 Abstract 4078. . Retrieved 11 January 2010.

[9] Varma, N.; et al. (August 30, 2009). "Efficiency of calendar based ICD checks: conventional follow-up compared to remote monitoring in the TRUST trial" (http://spo.escardio.org/abstract-book/presentation.aspx?id=67474). Barcelona, Spain: ESC Congress. pp. Abstract 86114. . Retrieved 11 January 2010.

[10] Varma, N.; et al. (August 31, 2009). "Event notification by remote monitoring systems performing automatic daily checks: load, characteristics and clinical utility" (http://spo.escardio.org/abstract-book/presentation.aspx?id=67579). Barcelona, Spain: ESC Congress. pp. Abstract 87438. . Retrieved 11 January 2010.

[11] "Our History" (http://www.biotronik.com/portal/4595). Biotronik. . Retrieved 12 January 2010.

[12] Versweyveld, Leslie (23 October 2001). "Two U.S. hospitals implant first BIOTRONIK pacemakers with Home Monitoring Technology" (http://www.hoise.com/vmw/01/articles/vmw/LV-VM-11-01-15.html). Virtual Medical Worlds Monthly. . Retrieved 12 January 2010.

[13] "OBIT/BIOTRONIK -- Professor Dr. Max Schaldach" (http://www.allbusiness.com/company-activities-management/company-structures/6070009-1.html). *Business Wire*. All Business.com. 7 May 2001. . Retrieved 12 January 2010.

[14] "BIOTRONIK Forges Ahead Toward Medtech Leadership Position" (http://findarticles.com/p/articles/mi_m0EIN/is_2008_Sept_1/ai_n28047799/?tag=col1;co-competitors). *Business Wire*. BNET CBS Interactive. 1 Sept 2008. . Retrieved 12 January 2010.
[15] "Nominated for the German Federal President's "Deutscher Zukunftspreis" (German Future Award): BIOTRONIK Home Monitoring for Online Monitoring of Heart Patients" (http://www.reuters.com/article/idUS107222+28-Sep-2009+BW20090928). Reuters. 28 Sept. 2009. . Retrieved 12 January 2010.

Telemental_Health

Telemental Health is the use of telecommunications technology to provide mental health services to individuals in communities or locations that are underserviced, typically as a result of geographic isolation. Examples of telemental health services include providing health workers in remote areas with continuing education on mental health topics, videoconferenced consultations on routine and urgent mental health cases using a "virtual" case management team, and providing direct mental health care services through two-way interactive systems. One of the most controversial telemental health care applications is providing treatment services over the Internet directly which, while showing early promise, will likely require considerable development to be made practical.

While telecommunications have been used for decades to provide some mental health services (usually on an emergency basis or for experimental purposes), it was only in the 1990s that telemental health care services truly came into their own. Despite the early success of telemental health care services however, wide-scale implementation remains dependent on policy and funding initiatives although the outlook remains positive.

External links

- Telemental Health Guide [1]

See also

- Telehealth
- Telemedicine

References

[1] http://www.tmhguide.org

Telenursing

Telenursing refers to the use of telecommunications and information technology for providing nursing services in health care whenever a large physical distance exists between patient and nurse, or between any number of nurses. As a field it is part of telehealth, and has many points of contacts with other medical and non-medical applications, such as telediagnosis, teleconsultation, telemonitoring, etc.

Telenursing is achieving a large rate of growth in many countries, due to several factors: the preoccupation in driving down the costs of health care, an increase in the number of aging and chronically ill population, and the increase in coverage of health care to distant, rural, small or sparsely populated regions. Among its many benefits, telenursing may help solve increasing shortages of nurses; to reduce distances and save travel time, and to keep patients out of hospital. A greater degree of job satisfaction has been registered among telenurses.[1]

Applications

One of the most distinctive telenursing applications is home care. For example, patients who are immobilized, or live in remote or difficult to reach places, citizens who have chronic ailments, such as chronic obstructive pulmonary disease, diabetes, congestive heart disease, or disabilitating diseases, such as neural degenerative diseases (Parkinson's disease, Alzheimer's disease, ALS), etc., may stay at home and be "visited" and assisted regularly by a nurse via videoconferencing, internet, videophone, etc. Still other applications of home care are the care of patients in immediate post-surgical situations, the care of wounds, ostomies, handicapped individuals, etc. In normal home health care, one nurse is able to visit up to 5-7 patients per day. Using telenursing, one nurse can “visit” 12-16 patients in the same amount of time. [Needs source]

A common application of telenursing is also used by call centers operated by managed care organizations, which are staffed by registered nurses who act as case managers or perform patient triage, information and counseling as a means of regulating patient access and flow and decrease the use of emergency rooms.

Telenursing can also involve other activities such as patient education, nursing teleconsultations, examination of results of medical tests and exams, and assistance to physicians in the implementation of medical treatment protocols.

Legal, ethical and regulatory issues

Telenursing is fraught with legal, ethical and regulatory issues, as it happens with telehealth as a whole. In many countries, interstate and intercountry practice of telenursing is forbidden (the attending nurse must have a license both in her state/country of residence and in the state/country where the patient receiving telecare is located). Legal issues such as accountability and malpractice, etc. are also still largely unsolved and difficult to address.

In addition, there are many considerations related to patient confidentiality and safety of clinical data.

See also

- telephone triage

References

Notes

[1] Nurses Happier Using Telecare, Says International Survey (http://www.e-health-insider.com/news/item.cfm?ID=1263), eHealth Insider website, 15 June 2005, retrieved 2009-04-04;

Bibliography

- *Telenursing: Nursing Practice in Cyberspace.* By Charles C Sharpe, 2000. 280 pg.
- *Textbook in Health Informatics: A Nursing Perspective.* Edited by J. Mantas, A. Hasman, 2002. IOS Press, 504 pg.
- *International Standards for Telenursing Programmes*, International Council of Nurses, 2001. 40 pg. (http://www.icn.ch/bookshop.htm)

External links

- Post discharge follow-up calls (http://www.telenursefirst.com/). TeleNurse First.
- Telenursing (http://www.allhealthnet.com/Nursing/Telenursing/). AllHealth.net
- Telehealth: Issues for Nursing (http://www.ana.org/readroom/tele2.htm). American Nursing Association.
- New nursing technologies: What you need to know (http://www.findarticles.com/p/articles/mi_qa3689/is_199708/ai_n8760283). By Simpson, Roy L. *Nursing*. August 1997.
- Telehome Care Clinical Guidelines^ (http://www.atmeda.org/news/list.html). American Telemedicine Association.
- Telenursing and Licensure (http://www.bne.state.tx.us/telenurse.htm). Board of Nursing Examiners.
- Interstate Licensure for Telenursing (http://tie.telemed.org/articles/article.asp?path=articles&article=telenursingLicensure_gw_tie02.xml). By Glenn W. Wachter, May, 2002. TIE.
- Telehealth: Are you at risk? (http://www.afip.org/Departments/legalmed/jnrm2002/georgia.htm) By Georgia A. Martin. Nursing Risk Management 2002. AFIP.
- Telemedicine Applications in Telenursing 2003 (http://www.atmeda.org/news/selected2004.htm#nursing) and Telemedicine Applications in Telenursing 2004 (http://www.atmeda.org/news/selected2003.htm#nursing). Powerpoint presentations during the Annual Conference of the American Telemedicine Association.
- Telenursing Fact Sheet (http://www.icn.ch/matters_telenursing.htm). International Council of Nurses.
- Nurse Triage site specializing in personalized health information and support (http://www.healthcontactpartners.com/)
- The National Council of State Boards of Nursing Position Paper on Telenursing: A Challenge to Regulation (http://www.ncsbn.org/public/news/res/Telenursing Paper.pdf). The National Council of State Boards. August 1999.
- International Society for Telemedicine & eHealth (ISfTeH) (http://www.isft.net) - Telenursing Working Group

Telepathology

Not to be confused with the paranormal belief in telepathy.

Telepathology is the practice of pathology at a distance. It uses telecommunications technology to facilitate the transfer of image-rich pathology data between distant locations for the purposes of diagnosis, education, and research.[1] [2] Performance of telepathology requires that a pathologist selects the video images for analysis and the rendering diagnoses. The use of "television microscopy", the forerunner of telepathology, did not require that a pathologist have physical or virtual "hands-on" involvement in the selection of microscopic fields-of-view for analysis and diagnosis.

An academic pathologist, Ronald S. Weinstein M.D., coined the term "telepathology" in 1986. In an editorial in a medical journal, Weinstein outlined the actions that would be needed to create remote pathology diagnostic services.[3] He and his collaborators published the first scientific paper on robotic telepathology.[4] Weinstein was also granted the first U.S. patents for robotic telepathology systems and telepathology diagnostic networks.[5] Dr. Weinstein is known to many as the "father of telepathology".[6] In Norway, Eide and Nordrum implemented the first sustainable clinical telepathology service in 1989.[7] This is still in operation, decades later. A number of clinical telepathology services have benefited many thousands of patients in North America, Europe, and Asia.

Telepathology has been successfully used for many applications including the rendering histopathology tissue diagnoses at a distance, for education, and for research. Although digital pathology imaging, including virtual microscopy, is the mode of choice for telepathology services in developed countries, analog telepathology imaging is still used for patient services in some developing countries.

Types of telepathology systems

Telepathology systems are divided into three major types: static image-based systems, real-time systems, and virtual slide systems. Static image systems have the benefit of being the most reasonably priced and usable systems. They have the significant drawback in only being able to capture a selected subset of microscopic fields for off-site evaluation. Real-time robotic microscopy systems and virtual slides allow a consultant pathologist the opportunity to evaluate histopathology slides in their entirety, from a distance. With real-time systems, the consultant actively operates a robotically controlled motorized microscope located at a distant site—changing focus, illumination, magnification, and field of view—at will. Either an analog video camera or a digital video camera can be used for robotic microscopy. Another form of real-time microscopy involves utilizing a high resolution video camera mounted on a path lab microscope to send live digital video of a slide to a large computer monitor at the pathologist's remote location via encrypted store-and-forward software. An echo-cancelling microphone at each end of the video conference allows the pathologist to communicate with the person moving the slide under the microscope. Virtual slide systems utilize automated digital slide scanners that create a digital image file of an entire glass slide (whole slide image). This file is stored on a computer server and can be navigated at a distance, over the Internet, using a browser.[8] Digital imaging is required for virtual microscopy.

While real-time and virtual slide systems offer higher diagnostic accuracy when compared with static-image telepathology, there are drawbacks to each. Real-time systems perform best on local area networks (LANs), but performance may suffer if employed during periods of high network traffic or using the Internet proper as a backbone. Expense is an issue with real-time systems and virtual slide systems as they can be costly. Virtual slide telepathology is emerging as the technology of choice for telepathology services. However, high throughput virtual slide scanners (those producing one virtual slide or more per minute) are currently expensive. Also, virtual slide digital files are relatively large, often exceeding one gigabyte in size. Storing and simultaneously retrieving large numbers of telepathology whole-slide image files can be cumbersome, introducing their own workflow challenges in the clinical laboratory.

Uses and benefits of telepathology

Telepathology is currently being used for a wide spectrum of clinical applications including diagnosing of frozen section specimens[9] , primary histopathology diagnoses[10] , second opinion diagnoses[11] , subspecialty pathology expert diagnoses[12] , education[13] , compentency assessment[14] , and research. Benefits of telepathology include providing immediate access to off-site pathologists for rapid frozen section diagnoses. Another benefit can be gaining direct access to subspecialty pathologists such as a renal pathologist, a neuropathologist, or a dermatopathologist, for immediate consultations.

Telepathology services by country

Canada

Canada Health Infoway is the organization responsible for the implementation of telepathology in Canada. Canada Health Infoway is a federal non-profit which provides funding for improving digital health infrastructure.

Canada Health Infoway has targeted funding of $1.2 million CAD to the Telepathology Solution for the province of British Columbia.[15] The system is designed to connect all pathologists within the province. The long-term expectations are improvement to patient care and safety through access to pathology expertise, improved timeliness of results and quality of service.

In Ontario, the University Health Network (UHN) hospitals are the primary drivers of the development of telepathology. The three northern Ontario communities of Timmins, Sault Ste. Marie and Kapuskasing have several community hospitals virtually linked to UHN pathologists via the Internet 24 hours a day[16] .

See also

- Pathology
- Anatomical Pathology
- Cytopathology
- Digital pathology
- Microscopy
- Medical laboratory
- Virtual microscope
- Virtual slide

References

[1] Weinstein, RS; Graham, AM; Richter, LC; Barker, GP; Krupinski, EA; Lopez, AM; Yagi, Y; Gilbertson, JR et al. (2009), "Overview of telepathology, virtual microscopy and whole slide imagining: Prospects for the future.", *Hum Pathol* **40**: 1057–1069

[2] Kumar, S (2009), Kumar S, Dunn BE (editors), ed., "Telepathology: An Audit", *In: Telepathology* (Springer-Verlag Berlin Heidelberg): 225–229

[3] Weinstein, RS (1986), "Prospects for telepatholgy (Editorial)", *Hum Pathol* **17**: 443-434

[4] Weinstein, RS; Bloom, KJ (1987), "Telepathology and the networking of pathology diagnostic services.", *Arch Path Lab Med* **111**: 646–652

[5] Kayser, K; Szymas, J; Weinstein (1999), "Telepathology: Telecommunications, Electronic Education and Publication in Pathology", *Springer, NY*: 1–186

[6] http://www.union.edu/N/DS/s.php?s=8942

[7] Nordrum, I; Engum, B; Rinde, E`; *et al* (1991), "Remote frozen section service: A telepathology project to northern Norway.", *Hum Pathol* **1991**: 514–518

[8] Kayser, K; Molnar, B; Weinstein, RS, "Digital pathology virtual slide technology in tissue-based diagnosis, research and education.", *VSV Interdisciplinary Medical Publishing* (Berlin): 1–193

[9] Evans, AJ; Chetty, R; Clarke, BA; Croul, S; Ghazarian; Kiehl, TR; Ordonez, BP; Ilaalagan, S et al., "Primary frozen section diagnosis by robotic microscopy and virtual slide telepathology: the University Health Network experience.", *Hum Pathol* **40**: 1069–1081

[10] Dunn, BE; Choi, H; Recla, DL; Kerr, SE; Wagenman, BL, "Robotic surgical telepathology between the Iron Mountain and Milwaukee Department of Veterans Affairs Medical Centers: a 12-year experience.", *Hum Pathol* **40**: 1092–1099

[11] Graham, AR; Bhattacharyya, AK; Scott, KM; Lian, F; Grasso, LL; Richter, LC; Henderson, JT; Carpenter, JB et al., "Virtual slide telepatholgoy for an academic teaching hospital surgical patholgoy quality assurance program.", *Hum Pathol* **40**: 1129–1136

[12] Massone, C; Soyer, HP; Lozzi, GP; DiStefani, A; Leinweber, B; Gabler, G; et al, "Feasibility and diagnostic agreement in teledermatology using a virtual slide system", *Hum Pathol* **38**: 546–554

[13] Dee, FR (2009), "Virtual microscopy in pathology education", *Hum Pathol* **40**: 1112–1121

[14] Bruch, LA; De Young, BR; Kreiter, CD; Haugen, TH; Leaven, TC; Dee, FR (2009), "Competency assessment of residents in surgical pathology using virtual microscopy.", *Hum Pathol* **40**: 1122–1128

[15] *Information Resource Management Plan 2007/08* (http://www.health.gov.bc.ca/library/publications/annualrpts/irmp/IRMP_07_08_web.pdf), British Columbia Ministry of Health Knowledge Management and Technology Division, , retrieved November 23, 2011

[16] "UHN establishes first telepathology system in Ontario" (https://www.infoway-inforoute.ca/lang-en/about-infoway/news/news-releases/613-uhn-establishes-first-telepathology-system-in-ontario), *News Releases* (Canada Health Infoway), , retrieved November 23, 2011

Bibliography

- Cross SS, Dennis T, Start RD. Telepathology: current status and future prospects in diagnostic histopathology. Histopathology 2002; 41:91-109.
- Della Mea V, Beltrami CA. Current experiences with internet telepathology and possible evolution in the next generation of Internet services. Anal Cell Pathol 2000; 21:127-34.
- Frierson HF Jr, Galgano MT. Frozen-section diagnosis by wireless telepathology and ultra portable computer: use in pathology resident/faculty consultation. Hum Pathol 2007; 38:1330-4.
- Halliday BE, Bhattacharyya AK, Graham AR, et al. Diagnostic accuracy of an international static-imaging telepathology consultation service. Hum Pathol 1997; 28:17-21.
- Kaplan KJ, Burgess JR, Sandberg GD, et al. Use of robotic telepathology for frozen-section diagnosis: a retrospective trial of a telepathology system for intraoperative consultation. Mod Pathol 2002; 15:1197–1204.
- Krupinski E, Weinstein RS, Bloom KJ, Rozek LS. Progress in telepathology: System implementation and testing. Advances in Path Lab Med 1993; 6:63-87.
- Krupinski EA. Virtual slide telepathology workstation-of-the-future: lessons learned from teleradiology. Semin Diagn Pathol 2009; 26:194-205.
- Leung ST, Kaplan KJ. Medicolegal aspects of telepathology. Hum Pathol 2009; 40:1137-1142.
- Maiolino P, De Vico G. Telepathology in veterinary diagnostic cytopathology. In: Kumar S, Dunn BE, editors. Telepathology. Berlin, Springer, 2009; 6:63-69.
- Nordrum I, Eide TJ. Remote frozen section service in Norway. Arch Anat Cytol Pathol 1995; 43:253-256.
- O'Malley DP. Practical applications of telepathology using morphology-based anatomic pathology. Arch Pathol Lab Med 2008; 132:743-4.
- Schroeder JA. Ultrasructural telepathology: remote EM diagnostic via Internet. In: Kumar S, Dunn BE, editors. Telepathology. Berlin, Springer, 2009; 14:179-204.
- Sinard JH. Practical pathology informatics. New York, Springer. 2006:265-286.
- Weinstein RS: Prospects for telepathology. (Editorial), Human Path 1986; 17:433 434.
- Weinstein RS, Bhattacharyya AK, Graham AR, et al. Telepathology: a ten-year progress report. Hum Pathol 1997;28:1–7.
- Weinstein RS, Bloom KJ, Rozek LS: Telepathology and the networking of pathology diagnostic services. Arch Path Lab Med 1987; 111:646-652.
- Weinstein RS, Descour MR, Liang C, et al. Telepathology overview: from concept to implementation. Hum Pathol 2001; 32:1283-99.

- Weinstein RS, Graham AM, Richter LC, Barker GP, Krupinski EA, Lopez AM, Erps KA, Yagi Y, Gilbertson JR, Bhattacharyya AK. Overview of telepathology, virtual microscopy and whole slide imagining: Prospects for the future. Hum Pathol, 2009; 40: 1057-1069.
- Williams S, Henricks WH, Becich MJ, et al. Telepathology for patient care: what am I getting myself into? Adv Anat Pathol 2010; 17:130-49.

External links

Informative sites or links

- Accelpath - Accelerated Digital Telepathology - Digital Pathology and Telepathology solutions (http://www.AccelPath.com/)
- APIII (http://www.pathinformatics.pitt.edu/) (a national pathology informatics meeting's website with archived presentations and contact information for faculty)
- Pathology Visions (http://www.pathologyvisions.com/index.html) (a national digital pathology conference)
- Association for Pathology Informatics (http://www.pathologyinformatics.org/)
- Digital Pathology Association (http://www.digitalpathologyassociation.org/)
- Digital Pathology Blog (http://www.tissuepathology.typepad.com/)
- American Telemedicine Association (http://www.americantelemed.org/i4a/pages/index.cfm?pageid=1)
- College of American Pathologists (http://www.cap.org/apps/cap.portal)
- United States and Canadian Academy of Pathology (http://www.uscap.org/home.htm)

Links to articles

- New Developments in Digital Pathology: from Telepathology to Virtual Pathology Laboratory (http://iospress.metapress.com/content/hgjhbq80evk7x8un/)
- Feeding OWL: Extracting and Representing the Content of Pathology Reports (http://acl.ldc.upenn.edu/W/W04/W04-0607.pdf)
- Organizing Knowledge in a Semantic Web for Pathology (http://www.springerlink.com/content/17k5vbjjawljmrd7/)
- Digital medicine in the virtual hospital of the future

Academic digital pathology sites

- Welcome to Digital Pathology at Brown Medical School (http://www.brown.edu/Courses/Digital_Path/)
- Holycross Cancer Center (Poland, Kielce) Pathomorphology Department virtual slides (http://www.telepatologia.onkol.kielce.pl/index.php?page=wszystkie_slajdy)
- Digital Pathology Imaging Group at University of Pittsburgh Medical Center (http://telepathology.upmc.edu/)

Other relevant sites

- Digital pathology: DICOM-conform draft, testbed, and first results (http://portal.acm.org/citation.cfm?id=1282562.1282636&jmp=cit&coll=GUIDE&dl=GUIDE&CFID=72380999&CFTOKEN=86827451#CIT/)
- Guidon Blog on whole slide image analysis (http://www.flagshipbio.com/blog/)
- OpenSlide - C library that provides a simple interface to read whole-slide images (http://openslide.cs.cmu.edu/).

Telephone_triage

Telephone triage is defined as the management of patient health concerns and symptoms via a telephone interaction (telecommunications) by "advice nurses". It is thus an aspect of telenursing. It can also be considered an aspect of telemedicine and telehealth utilizing an older form of technology (telephone lines). Telehealth is defined as the delivery of health related services and information via telecommunications technologies and is now the umbrella term describing all the possible variations of healthcare services using telecommunications.

Uses of Telephone Triage

Triage means a sorting out. Telephone triage nurses utilize protocols or guidelines, in paper or electronic format to help sort symptoms, from "chest pain to chicken pox". Telephone triage involves ranking clients' health problems according to their urgency, educating and advising clients, and making safe, effective, and appropriate dispositions—all by telephone. It may include everything from disease management, AIDS counseling and child abuse hotlines to 911 and telemetry monitoring, and takes place in settings as diverse as emergency rooms, large call centers and hospices.

Telephone triage nurses have a range of titles: "advice nurses", "telepractitioners", "telenurses", "telepractice nurses" or "consulting nurses". In one 8-hour shift, a telenurse may field 60-80 telephone calls—one every 6 – 10 minutes—painstakingly assessing headaches, newborn rashes, chest pain, possible allergic reactions, medication questions, and seasonal flu and fevers. Nurses may also direct clients to obtain a second medical opinion, or advise them where to find relevant, current health information. They might counsel or perform crisis intervention for a threatened suicide. What was traditionally done informally in emergency rooms, clinics, and physicians' offices for years has evolved into a new nursing subspecialty called telephone triage.

Telenurses practice in a range of settings, from large medical call centers, physician's offices, clinics, hospices, college health centers, disease management call centers, poison centers, and emergency departments.

Research on Telenurse Decision-making

Telephone triage — the safe, effective and appropriate disposition of health related problems by RNs — always involves "decision-making under conditions of uncertainty and urgency." (Patel, 1996) "Uncertainty" because decisions are often made based on partial or inaccurate information; "urgency" because calls must be processed within a brief time frame — usually 6–10 minutes average. In new research, telephone triage has been compared to the work of air traffic controllers, EMDs and firefighters — all high stakes activities. Vimla Patel, Ph.D., described how a group of RNs working in an emergency department setting made "real world" decisions in telephone triage. She discovered that these nurses used pattern recognition, rules of thumb and context as major strategies to make decisions.

Protocols

Protocols or guidelines are essentially" standing orders" for nurses for the assessment and management of a range of symptoms. Protocols may be in paper or electronic format. Some developers see protocols as decision-making tools; others as decision support tools. This is an area of controversy in this new field.

The research on nurse decision-making by Patel and other experts has important implications for protocol design. The strategies of pattern recognition, rules of thumb and context should be incorporated into all elements of any decision support system as well as telenurse training and forms. The goal should be to mimic how the brain naturally solves problems in "real world" situations.

Telephone triage is a high-risk area of practice, primarily because nurses cannot see the patient with whom they are speaking. Thus, training and guidelines are essential to support the nurse. Relying on protocols to take the place of formal instruction can be a mistake, and over reliance on a decision-making tool can lead to mistriage.

Generally, experience and specialized training combined with strong decision support tools are the best approach to telepractice. Potential problems and misunderstandings can be averted through instruction in the correct and safe operation of the protocols and documentation form. gowri

Brief history

Informal telephone triage is as old as the telephone itself. In fact, one of the first calls made by Alexander Graham Bell was for assistance following a battery acid burn (Grumet, 1979). In the early days, physicians were quick to install telephones in their offices, seeing that these new tools could help their practices. Initially, physicians performed telephone advice. Telephone management has always comprised a large percentage of several physicians' practices – pediatrics, Women's Health and Family Practice specialties.

In the 1970s, several health maintenance organizations began utilizing nurses to give telephone advice—in the role that physicians once served. A wide variety of similar systems have sprung up over the last decade. In 1990, the term "telephone triage" appeared on Medline indexes—a formal acknowledgement of this new subspecialty.

Telephone triage formalization

In the early 70's, telephone triage had few job qualifications—most nurses were felt to be qualified. As the field evolved into a recognized subspecialty, managers discovered that the high-stakes, high stress work required seasoned RNs with many years of "bedside" decision-making experience. Thus, new graduates were not considered the best candidates for the task of telephone triage.

Certainly, there are exceptions to this rule. However, we know that less experience results in over triage (Patel, 1996), while increased experience results in more appropriate decisions. The new RN, with little or no bedside decision-making experience will require time to build up these skills. Whether in the clinic, office, hospital or in the emergency department setting, five to ten year's experience provides the foundation necessary for good decision making by phone—a considerably more difficult task.

RNs are considered the best choice not only because they are autonomous professionals, but they are also "the lowest paid person who can safely do the job" (Schmitt, 1980). Telephone triage requires excellence in interpersonal skill or "telephone charisma" (articulate, personable, resourceful, dedication to service). There must be a good match between the work—high volume, high-pressure decision making under conditions of uncertainty and urgent—and the practitioner's temperament—calm, mature and patient. Computer literacy is desirable.

Since the 70's most training was "on the job", essentially "see one, do one, teach one". Each new advice nurse had to learn through trial and error, essentially "reinventing the training wheel" with each new employee. In the 90's, formal training programs emerged. Currently, the best training programs have a minimum of 40 hours. Orientation addresses an overview of the field and the nursing role, the nursing process, communication aspects, history taking, interview and documentation skills, protocol use and medical legal aspects.

Two types of training and education currently exist—in-house and national conferences. In house trainers employ a variety of training methodologies, since research demonstrates that individuals learn differently and learning happens best when all senses are utilized. In-house training techniques include reading, lecture, discussion, "shadowing", written exercises in interview and documentation, audiotapes analysis/critique, preceptor programs and role-play of mock calls. Role-play is an excellent method to cumulatively integrate the new skills and tools (protocols and documentation form) and to simulate the actual task. Preceptors can support and counsel the new advice nurse in the first three to six months.

National conferences provide a broad perspective and opportunity to network and problem solves. Since 1994, conferences on telephone triage have provided a national forum for manager and practitioner alike to network and share experience and expertise. The final step in formal education will be accreditation—not yet a reality—but anticipated within the next five to ten years.

References

- Wheeler, S.Q, and Windt, J. (1993) Telephone Triage: Theory, Practice and Protocol Development, Delmar Thomson, Albany, NY.
- Wheeler, S.Q. (2003) Telephone Triage Protocols for Adult and School Age Populations with Women's Health and Infant/Child Protocols, Aspen Publishers, Gaithersburg, MD.
- Wheeler, S.Q. (2000) Telephone Triage: Past, Present and Future www.teletriage.com

Resources

- Post discharge follow up calls [1]. Telenurse First
- Teletriage consulting site by Sheila Wheeler [2]
- Teletriage consulting site by Carol Rutenberg [3]
- Association of Telehealth Service Providers [4]
- American Academy of Ambulatory Care Nursing (AACN) [5]
- Nurse Triage site specializing in personalized health information and support [6]

References

[1] http://www.telenursefirst.com/
[2] http://www.teletriage.com/
[3] http://www.telephone-triage.com/
[4] http://www.atsp.org/homepage.asp
[5] http://www.aaacn.org/
[6] http://www.healthcontactpartners.com/

Telepsychiatry

Telepsychiatry is the application of Telemedicine to the field of Psychiatry.

It has been the most successful of all the telemedicine applications so far, because of its need for only a good videoconferencing facility between the patient and the psychiatrist, especially for follow-up. There are sub-specialties like *forensic telepsychiatry*,[1] in which the patient is typically an inmate accessing the psychiatrist who is from a supporting institution, and *home-based telepsychiatry*,[2] whereby the patient is in his own home or office, accessing the physician via webcam and high-speed internet. Another common application is for patients in rural or underserved areas, and there are a large number of grass roots telepsychiatry programs springing up in the United States and elsewhere to address this problem. In the U.S., Medicare and the various state Medicaids, as well as nearly all private health insurance providers, pay equally for telepsychiatry as for face to face psychiatric medication management visits.[3]

A recent innovation is the development of the subspecialty of emergency psychiatry via telemedicine. Research is currently on-going to develop the unique guidelines required to provide consultation for emergency psychiatric patients such as the evaluation of the suicidal, homidical, violent, psychotic, depressed, manic, and acutely anxious patient.[4] Emergency telepsychiatry services are being provided to hospital emergency departments, jails, community mental health centers, substance abuse treatment facilities, and schools.[5]

References

[1] Jardine, Richard. "Forensic Telepsychiatry" (http://www.telepsychiatry.slam.nhs.uk/Home/ForensicTP/tabid/332/Default.aspx) (Electronic). . Retrieved 07-10-2010.

[2] "Treatment of Opioid Dependence via Home-Based Telepsychiatry - Ikelheimer 59 (10): 1218 - Psychiatr Serv" (http://psychservices.psychiatryonline.org/cgi/content/full/59/10/1218-a). Psychservices.psychiatryonline.org. doi:10.1176/appi.ps.59.10.1218-a. . Retrieved 2010-07-10.

[3] Surface, David (January/February 2007), "Country Comfort: Mental Health Telemedicine in Rural America", *Social Work* **7** (1): 28–31

[4] Shore JH, Hilty DM, Yellowlees P (2007). "Emergency management guidelines for telepsychiatry". *General Hospital Psychiatry* **29** (3): 199–206. doi:10.1016/j.genhosppsych.2007.01.013. PMC 1986661. PMID 17484936.

[5] "Telepsychiatry in the Emergency Department: Overview and Case Studies" (http://www.chcf.org/~/media/Files/PDF/T/TelepsychiatryProgramsED.pdf) (PDF). . Retrieved 2010-07-10.

Further reading

- Frueh BC, Monnier J, Elhai JD, Grubaugh AL, Knapp RG (2004). "Telepsychiatry treatment outcome research methodology: efficacy versus effectiveness". *Telemedicine Journal and E-health* **10** (4): 455–8. doi:10.1089/tmj.2004.10.455. PMID 15689650.
- Hilty DM, Marks SL, Urness D, Yellowlees PM, Nesbitt TS (January 2004). "Clinical and educational telepsychiatry applications: a review". *Canadian Journal of Psychiatry* **49** (1): 12–23. PMID 14763673.
- Frueh BC, Monnier J, Elhai JD, Grubaugh AL, Knapp RG (2004). "Telepsychiatry treatment outcome research methodology: efficacy versus effectiveness". *Telemedicine Journal and E-health* **10** (4): 455–8. doi:10.1089/tmj.2004.10.455. PMID 15689650.
- Monnier J, Knapp RG, Frueh BC (December 2003). "Recent advances in telepsychiatry: an updated review". *Psychiatric Services* **54** (12): 1604–9. doi:10.1176/appi.ps.54.12.1604. PMID 14645799.

External links

- Telemental Health Guide (http://www.tmhguide.org)
- http://www.cpa-apc.org/publications/archives/Bulletin/2003/october/hilty.asp A review on the effectiveness
- Some related links (http://telemed.org/europe/links/telepsych.asp)
- A feasibility study (http://www.telepsychiatry.slam.nhs.uk/Portals/9/douments/final.version.feasibility.08.03.doc)
- American Association for Emergency Psychiatry (http://emergencypsychiatry.org)
- (http://www.telelive.org)
- Voyager Telepsychiatry (http://www.telepsychiatry.com)
- JSA Health Telepsychiatry (http://www.jsahealthmd.com)

Teleradiology

Teleradiology is the transmission of radiological patient images, such as x-rays, CTs, and MRIs, from one location to another for the purposes of sharing studies with other radiologists and physicians. Teleradiology is a growth technology given that imaging procedures are growing approximately 15% annually against an increase of only 2% in the Radiologist population.

Teleradiology improves patient care by allowing Radiologists to provide services without actually having to be at the location of the patient. This is particularly important when a sub-specialist such as a MRI Radiologist, Neuroradiologist, Pediatric Radiologist, or Musculoskeletal Radiologist is needed, since these professionals are generally only located in large metropolitan areas working during day time hours. Teleradiology allows for trained specialists to be available 24/7.

Teleradiology utilizes standard network technologies such as the internet, telephone lines, wide area network, local area network (LAN) and the latest high tech being computer clouds. Specialized software is used to transmit the images and enable the Radiologist to effectively analyze what can be hundreds of images for a given study. Technologies such as advanced graphics processing, voice recognition, and image compression are often used in Teleradiology. Through Teleradiology, images can be sent to another part of the hospital, or to other locations around the world.

Reports

Teleradiologists can provide a Preliminary Read for emergency room cases and other emergent cases or a Final Read for the official patient record and for use in billing.

Preliminary Reports include all pertinent findings and a phone call for any critical findings. For some Teleradiology services, the turnaround time is extremely rapid with a 30 minute standard turnaround and expedited for critical and stroke studies.

Teleradiology Final Reports can be provided for emergent and non-emergent studies. Final reports include all findings and require access to prior studies and all relevant patient information for a complete diagnosis. Phone calls with any critical findings are signs of quality services.

Teleradiology Preliminary or Final Reports can be provided for all doctors and hospitals overflow studies. Teleradiology can be available for intermittent coverage as an extension of practices and will provide patients with the highest quality care.

Subspecialties

Some teleradiologists are fellowship trained and have a wide variety of subspecialty expertise including such difficult-to-find areas as Neuroradiology, Pediatric Neuroradiology, Musculo-skeletal MRI, Mammography, Nuclear Cardiology.

Regulations

In the United States, Medicare and Medicaid laws require the Teleradiologist to be on U.S. soil in order to qualify for reimbursement of the Final Read.

In addition, advanced teleradiology systems must also be HIPAA compliant, which helps to ensure patients' privacy. HIPAA (Health Insurance Portability and Accountability Act of 1996) is a uniform, federal floor of privacy protections for consumers. It limits the ways that entities can use patients' personal information and protects the privacy of all medical information no matter what form it is in. Quality teleradiology must abide by important HIPAA rules to ensure patients' privacy is protected.

Also State laws governing the licensing requirements and medical malpractice insurance coverage required for physicians vary from state to state. Ensuring compliance with these laws is a significant overhead expense for larger multi-state teleradiology groups.

Industry growth

Until the late 1990s teleradiology was primarily used by individual radiologists to interpret occasional emergency studies from offsite locations, often in the radiologists home. The connections were made through standard analog phone lines.

Teleradiology expanded rapidly as the growth of the internet and broad band combined with new CT scanner technology to become an essential tool in trauma cases in emergency rooms throughout the country. The occasional 2-3 x ray studies a week soon became 3-10 CT scans, or more, a night. Because ER physicians are not trained to read CT scans or MRI's, radiologists went from working 8–10 hours a day, five and half days a week to a schedule of 24 hours a day, 7 days a week coverage. This became a particularly acute challenge in smaller rural facilities that only had one solo radiologist with no other to share call.

These circumstances spawned a post dot.com boom of firms and groups that provided outsourced, off-site teleradiology on-call services to hospitals and Radiology Groups around the country. As an example, a teleradiology firm might cover trauma at a hospital in Indiana with doctors based in Texas. Some firms even used overseas doctors in locations like Australia and India. Nighthawk, founded by Dr. Paul Berger, was the first to station U.S. licensed radiologists overseas (initially Australia and later Switzerland) to maximize the time zone difference to provide nightcall in U.S. hospitals.

The early innovators in this field like Teleradiology Solutions, Nighthawk Radiology, The Radlinx Group, and Virtual Radiology Consultants (VRC or VRN most recently), became multi million dollar companies today. Nighthawk (symbol: NHWK) and VRC (symbol: VRAD) ultimately went public and established almost a billion dollars in market capitalization.

However, on May 17, 2010, Providence Equity Partners acquired and took private Virtual Radiologic.[1] Moreover, on September, 27, 2010, Virtual Radiologic and NightHawk Radiology Announced their Merger.[2] Finally, on December 23, 2010, Virtual Radiologic (vRad) and NightHawk Radiology announced the completion of their previously announced merger, with NightHawk continuing as a wholly owned subsidiary of vRad. [3]

The Radlinx Group, founded by Greg Lowenstein and Mark Bakken, pioneered the expansion of teleradiology services beyond just night coverage to also provide coverage to hundreds of small rural hospitals and clinics, throughout the U.S., who otherwise had no on-site access to full-time radiologists.

Currently teleradiology firms are facing pricing pressures. Industry consolidation is likely as there are more than 500 of these firms, large and small, throughout the United States.

See also

- Telemedicine
- PACS
- DICOM

References

[1] "Providence to Take Virtual Radiologic Private." (http://dealbook.nytimes.com/2010/05/17/providence-to-take-virtual-radiologic-private/). New York Times. 2010-05-17. .

[2] "Virtual Radiologic and NightHawk Radiology Announced a Merger." (http://www.prnewswire.com/news-releases/virtual-radiologic-and-nighthawk-radiology-announce-merger-103849613.html). PR Newswire. 2010-09-27. .

[3] "VRad and Nighthawk Radiology Complete Merger." (http://www.itnonline.net/node/38565/3/). Imaging Technology News. 2010-12-23. .

Telerehabilitation

Telerehabilitation (or *e-rehabilitation*[1] [2]) is the delivery of rehabilitation services over telecommunication networks and the internet. Most types of services fall into two categories: clinical assessment (the patient's functional abilities in his or her environment), and clinical therapy. Some fields of rehabilitation practice that have explored telerehabilitation are: neuropsychology, speech-language pathology, audiology, occupational therapy, and physical therapy. Telerehabilitation can deliver therapy to people who cannot travel to a clinic because the patient has a disability or because of travel time. Telerehabilitation also allows experts in rehabilitation to engage in a clinical consultation at a distance.

Most telerehabilitation is highly visual. As of 2006 the most commonly used modalities are via webcams, videoconferencing, phone lines, videophones and webpages containing rich Internet applications. The visual nature of telerehabilitation technology limits the types of rehabilitation services that can be provided. It is most widely used for neuropsychological rehabilitation; fitting of rehabilitation equipment such as wheelchairs, braces or artificial limbs; and in speech-language pathology. Rich internet applications for neuropsychological rehabilitation (aka cognitive rehabilitation) of cognitive impairment (from many etiologies) was first introduced in 2001. This endeavor has recently (2006) expanded as a teletherapy application for cognitive skills enhancement programs for school children. Tele-audiology (hearing assessments) is a growing application. As of 2006, telerehabilitation in the practice of occupational therapy and physical therapy are very limited, perhaps because these two disciplines are more "hands on".

Two important areas of telerehabilitation research are (1) demonstrating equivalence of assessment and therapy to in-person assessment and therapy, and (2) building new data collection systems to digitize information that a therapist can use in practice. Ground-breaking research in telehaptics (the sense of touch) and virtual reality may broaden the scope of telerehabilitation practice, in the future.

In the United States, the National Institute on Disability and Rehabilitation Research's (NIDRR) [16] supports research and the development of telerehabilitation. NIDRR's grantees include the "Rehabilitation Engineering and Research Center" (RERC) at the University of Pittsburgh, the Rehabilitation Institute of Chicago, the State University of New York at Buffalo, and the National Rehabilitation Hospital in Washington DC. Other federal funders of research are the Veterans Administration, the Health Services Research Administration in the US Department of Health and Human Services, and the Department of Defense. Outside the United States, excellent research is conducted in Australia and Europe.

As of 2006, only a few health insurers in the United States will reimburse for telerehabilitation services. If the research shows that tele-assessments and tele-therapy are equivalent to clinical encounters, it is more likely that insurers and Medicare will cover telerehabilitation services.

History

In 1999, D.M. Angaran published "Telemedicine and Telepharmacy: Current Status and Future Implications" in the American Journal of Health-System Pharmacy. He provided a comprehensive history of telecommunications, the internet and telemedicine since the 1950s. The Department of Defense (DoD) and the National Aeronautics and Space Administration (NASA) spearheaded the technology in the United States during the Vietnam War and the space program; both agencies continue to fund advances in telemedicine.

Three early adopters of telemedicine were state penitentiary systems, rural health care systems, and the radiology profession. Telemedicine makes business sense for the states because they do not have to pay for security escorts to have a prisoner receive care outside the prison.

Rural telemedicine in the United States is heavily subsidized through federal agency grants for telecommunications operations. Most of this funding comes through the Health Services Research Administration and the Department of Commerce. Some state universities have obtained state funding to operate tele-clinics in rural areas. As of 2006, few (if any) of these programs are known to financially break-even, mostly because the Medicare program for people over age 65 (the largest payer) is very restrictive about paying for telehealth.

In contrast, the Veterans Administration is relatively active in using telemedicine for people with disabilities. There are several programs that provide annual physical exams or monitoring and consultation for veterans with spinal cord injuries. Similarly, some state Medicaid programs (for poor people and people with disabilities) have pilot programs using telecommunications to connect rural practitioners with subspecialty therapists. A few school districts in Oklahoma and Hawaii offer school-based rehabilitation therapy using therapy assistants who are directed by a remote therapist. The National Rehabilitation Hospital in Washington DC and Sister Kenny Rehabilitation Institute in Minneapolis provided assessment and evaluations to patients living in Guam and American Samoa. Cases included post-stroke, post-polio, autism, and wheel-chair fitting.

An argument can be made that "telerehabilitation" began in 1998 when NIDRR funded the first RERC on tele-rehabilitation. It was awarded to a consortium of biomedical engineering departments at the National Rehabilitation Hospital and The Catholic University of America, both located in Washington, DC; the Sister Kenny Rehabilitation Institute in Minnesota; and the East Carolina University in North Carolina. Some of this early research work, and its motivation, is reviewed in Winters (2002). The State of Science Conference held in 2002 convened most of military and civilian clinicians, engineers, and government officials interested in using telecommunications as a modality for rehabilitation assessment and therapy; a summary is provided in Rosen, Winters & Lauderdale (2002). The conference was attended by the incoming president of the American Telemedicine Association (ATA). This led to an invitation by ATA to the conference attendees to form a special interest group on telerehabilitation. NIDRR funded the second 5-year RERC on telerehabilitation in 2004, awarding it to the University of Pittsburgh. This RERC was renewed in 2010.

In 2001, O. Bracy, a neuropsychologist, introduced the first web based, rich internet application, for the telerehabilitation presentation of cognitive rehabilitation therapy. This system first provides the subscriber clinician with an economical means of treating their own patients over the internet. Secondly, the system then provides, directly to the patient, the therapy prescription set up and controlled by the member clinician. All applications and response data are transported via the internet in real time. The patient can login to do their therapy from home, the library or anywhere they have access to an internet computer. In 2006, this system formed the basis of a new system designed as a cognitive skills enhancement program for school children. Individual children or whole classrooms can participate in this program over the internet.

In 2006, M.J. McCue and S.E. Palsbo published an article in the Journal of Telemedicine and Telecare that explored how telemedicine can become a profitable business for hospitals. They argue that telerehabilitation should be expanded so that people with disabilities and people in pain (perhaps after hip-replacement surgery or people with arthritis) can get the rehabilitative therapy they need. It is unethical to limit paymente for telerehabilitation services only to patients in rural areas.

Research in telerehabilitation is in its infancy, with only a handful of equivalence trials. As of 2006, most peer-reviewed research in telemedicine are case reports of pilot programs or new equipment. Rehabilitation researchers need to conduct many more controlled experiments and present the evidence to clinicians (and payers) that telerehabilitation is clinically effective. The discipline of speech-language pathology is far head of occupational therapy and physical therapy in demonstrating equivalence over various types of telecommunications equipment.

Technologies

1. Plain old telephone service (POTS) with videophones/Phones in telerehabilitation

   There are several types of connections used with real time exchanges. Plain old telephone service (POTS) uses standard analog telephone lines. Videophones are used with POTS lines and include a camera, display screen, and telephone. Videophones use telephone lines that are available in most homes, so are easy to set up; however small display screens make them problematic for individuals with vision problems. This can be solved by using a large screen or television as a screen.
2. Videotelephony/Videotelephony in telerehabilitation

   The use of improved quality video-assisted telecommunication devices, such as videoconferencing, webcams and telepresence to assist in treatments.
3. Virtual reality/Virtual reality in telerehabilitation

   Virtual reality in telerehabilitation is one of the newest tools available in that area. This computer technology allows the development of three-dimensional virtual environments.
4. Motion technology/Motion technology in telerehabilitation
5. Web-based approaches/Web-based approaches in telerehabilitation

   Applications that run over the internet, just as if they were installed in your computer (called Rich Internet Applications), represent a new direction in software development. A person subscribes to the website rather than purchase the software. Any updates or changes to the software system are instantly available to all subscribers. The applications can be accessed from any location where one has access to an internet connected computer. Likewise, a patient's data is accessible from where ever the therapist is located. Neither the application nor the patient's data is tied to one computer.
6. Sensors and body monitoring/Sensors and body monitoring in telerehabilitation
7. Haptic technology/Haptic technology in telerehabilitation
8. Artificial intelligence/Artificial intelligence in telerehabilitation
9. Wireless technology/Wireless technology in telerehabilitation
10. PDAs/PDA in telerehabilitation
11. Mobile telephony/Mobile telephony in telerehabilitation
12. Electronic medical records/Electronic medical record telerehabilitation

Clinical applications of telerehabilitation

1. Review of telerehabilitation research on clinical populations
2. Professional to professional (clinic to clinic applications)
3. Telehealth – Information access
4. Clinical approaches
    1. Assessment
    2. Monitoring
    3. Intervention
    4. Telesupervision (of licensed assistants)
    5. Telementoring
    6. Tele-education
    7. Telementoring

Speech-language pathology

The clinical services provided by speech-language pathology readily lend themselves to telerehabilitation applications due to the emphasis on auditory and visual communicative interaction between the client and the clinician. As a result, the number of telerehabilitation applications in speech-language pathology tend to outnumber those in other allied health professions. To date, applications have been developed to assess and/or treat acquired adult speech and language disorders, stuttering, voice disorders, speech disorders in children, and swallowing dysfunction. The technology involved in these applications has ranged from the simple telephone (Plain Old Telephone System – POTS) to the use of dedicated Internet-based videoconferencing systems.

Early applications to assess and treat acquired adult speech and language disorders involved the use of the telephone to treat patients with aphasia and motor speech disorders (Vaughan, 1976, Wertz, et al., 1987), a computer controlled video laserdisc over the telephone and a closed-circuit television system to assess speech and language disorders (Wertz et al, 1987), and a satellite-based videoconferencing system to assess patients in rural areas (Duffy, Werven & Aronson, 1997). More recent applications have involved the use of sophisticated Internet-based videoconferencing systems with dedicated software which enable the assessment of language disorders (Georgeadis, Brennan, Barker, & Baron, 2004, Brennan, Georgeadis, Baron & Barker, 2004) and the assessment and treatment of motor speech disorders (Hill, Theodoros, Russell, Cahill, Ward, Clark, 2006; Theodoros, Constantinescu, Russell, Ward, Wilson & Wootton, in press) following brain impairment and Parkinson's disease. Collectively, these studies have revealed positive treatment outcomes, while assessment and diagnoses have been found to be comparable to face-to-face evaluations.

The treatment of stuttering has been adapted to a telerehabilitation environment with notable success. Two Australian studies (Harrison, Wilson & Onslow, 1999; Wilson, Onslow & Lincoln, 2004) involving the distance delivery of the Lidcombe program to children who stutter have utilized the telephone in conjunction with offline video recordings to successfully treat several children. Overall, the parents and children responded positively to the program delivered at a distant. Using a high speed videoconferencing system link, Sicotte, Lehoux, Fortier-Blanc and Leblanc (2003) assessed and treated six children and adolescents with a positive reduction in the frequency of dysfluency that was maintained six months later. In addition, a videoconferencing platform has been used successfully to provide follow-up treatment to an adult who had previously received intensive therapy (Kully, 200).

Reports of telerehabilitation applications in paediatric speech and language disorders are sparse. A recent Australian pilot study has investigated the feasibility of an Internet-based assessment of speech disorder in six children (Waite, Cahill, Theodoros, Russell, Busuttin, in press). High levels of agreement between the online and face-to-face clinicians for single-word articulation, speech intelligibility, and oro-motor tasks were obtained suggesting that the Internet-based protocol had the potential to be a reliable method for assessing paediatric speech disorders.

Voice therapy across a variety of types of voice disorders has been shown to be effectively delivered via a telerehabilitation application. Mashima et al. (2003) using PC based videoconferencing and speech analysis software compared 23 patients treated online with 28 persons treated face-to-face. The authors reported positive post treatment results with no significant difference in measures between the traditional and videoconferencing group, suggesting that the majority of traditional voice therapy techniques can be applied to distance treatment.

Although obvious limitations exist, telerehabilitation applications for the assessment of swallowing function have also been used with success. Lalor, Brown and Cranfield (2000) were able to obtain an initial assessment of the nature and extent of swallowing dysfunction in an adult via a videoconferencing link although a more complete evaluation was restricted due to the inability to physically determine the degree of laryngeal movement. A more sophisticated telerehabilitation application for the assessment of swallowing was developed by Perlman and Witthawaskul (2002) who described the use of real-time videofluoroscopic examination via the Internet. This system enabled the capture and display of images in real-time with only a three to five second delay.

There continues to be a need for ongoing research to develop and validate the use of telerehabilitation applications in speech-language pathology in a greater number and variety of adult and paediatric communication and swallowing disorders.

Disciplines and therapies

1. Speech-language pathology
2. Audiology
3. Physical therapy
4. Occupational therapy
5. Psychology
6. Nursing
7. Social work
8. Rehabilitation counseling/Vocational rehabilitation

Standards and training requirements

1. Telerehabilitation standards
2. Reimbursement policies/Reimbursement in telerehabilitation
3. Legislative activities/Legislative activities in telerehabilitation
4. Ethics and privacy issues/Ethics and privacy issues in telerehabilitation
5. Clinical and technology training issues

Related organizations

- American Telemedicine Association (ATA)
- American Speech-Language-Hearing Association (ASHA)
- Association of Telehealth Service Providers (ATSP)
- National Institute on Disability and Rehabilitation Research (NIDRR)
- Rehabilitation Engineering and Assistive Technology Society of North America (RESNA)
- Special Interest Group on Telerehabilitation (SIGOT)

See also

- Telemedicine
- Rehabilitation (neuropsychology)

References

[1] *E-health care information systems: an introduction for students and professionals*, John Wiley and Sons, 2005, p. 219, ISBN 9780787966188

[2] Lisa Keaton; Linda L. Pierce; Victoria Steiner; Karen Lance. "An E-rehabilitation Team Helps Caregivers Deal with Stroke" (http://ijahsp.nova.edu/articles/vol2num4/pierce-keaton.htm). *The Internet Journal of Allied Health Sciences and Practice* (Ijahsp.nova.edu) **2.4**. ISSN 1540-580X. . Retrieved 2011-03-26.

External links

Telerehabilitation (http://www.dmoz.org/Health/Medicine/Informatics/Telemedicine/Projects//) at the Open Directory Project

The_Continua_Health_Alliance

Continua HEALTH ALLIANCE	
Industry	Trade association
Founded	June 2006
Headquarters	Beaverton, Oregon, United States
Area served	Worldwide
Key people	Clint McClellan (President) Charles Parker (Executive Director)
Website	ContinuaAlliance.org [1]

Continua Health Alliance is an international non-profit, open industry group of nearly 240 healthcare providers, communications, medical, and fitness device companies.

Continua Health Alliance members aim to develop a system to deliver personal and individual healthcare.

Overview

Continua Health Alliance aims to establish a system of personal connected healthcare solutions. The goal of developing the solutions is to promote delivery of healthcare in the home providing independence, empowering individuals and providing the opportunity for truly personalized health and wellness management.[2]

Continua Health Alliance is working toward establishing systems of interoperable telehealth devices and services in three major categories: chronic disease management, aging independently, and health & physical fitness.

Continua members intend to create systems and devices for improving personal health. The technology platforms for these products and services are defined by the members and published in the Continua guidelines.

Devices and Services

Continua Health Alliance version 1 design guidelines are based on proven connectivity technical standards and include Bluetooth for wireless and USB for wired device connection. The group released the guidelines to the public in June 2009.[3]

The group is establishing a product certification program using its recognizable logo, the Continua Certified Logo program, signifying that the product is interoperable with other Continua-certified products. Products made under Continua Health Alliance guidelines will provide consumers with increased assurance of interoperability between devices, enabling them to more easily share information with caregivers and service providers.

Through collaborations with government agencies and other regulatory bodies, Continua works to provide guidelines for the effective management of diverse products and services from a global network of vendors.

Continua Alliance products make use of the ISO/IEEE 11073 Personal Health Data (PHD) Standards.

Major milestones and Status Information

Continua Health Alliance was founded on June 6, 2006[4]

Continua Health alliance performed its first public demonstration of interoperability on October 27, 2008 at the Partners Center for Connected Health 5th Annual Connected Health Symposium in Boston.[5]

Continua Health Alliance certified its first product [6], the Nonin 2500 PalmSAT handheld pulse oximeter with USB, on January 26, 2009.[7]

By the end of September 2010 there were fourteen certified products.[8]

Continua selected Bluetooth Low Energy and ZigBee wireless protocols as the wireless standards for its Version 2 Design Guidelines which are yet to be released. Bluetooth Low Energy is to be used for low-power mobile devices. ZigBee will be used for networked low-power sensors such as those enabling independent living.[9]

Members

Continua Health Alliance currently has nearly 240 member companies.[10]

Continua's Board of Directors is currently composed of the following companies:[11]

- Intel Corporation
- Roche Diagnostics
- Partners HealthCare
- Price Waterhouse Coopers
- Ascension Health
- CA, Inc.
- Cisco Systems
- Kaiser Permanente
- Medtronic
- Panasonic
- Philips
- Qualcomm
- Samsung Electronics
- Sharp

Organisational Structure

The Organisation is primarily staffed by volunteers from the member organisations that are organised in to working groups that address the goals of the alliance. Below the board of directors sit the following main working groups:[12]

- Global Policy Strategy Working Group
- Marketing Working Group
- Regulatory Working Group
- Technical Working Group
- Test & Certification Work Group - The Test and Certification Working Group is responsible for defining, implementing, and continuously improving the Test and Certification process and tools.
- Use Case Working Group
- Wellness Solutions Working Group

Relevant standards

- ISO/IEEE 11073
- ISO/IEEE 11073 Personal Health Data (PHD) Standards
- Bluetooth
- USB
- HL7
- Integrating the Healthcare Enterprise
- Zigbee

Website

The Continua Alliance website contains a full listing of member organisations, a directory of qualified products, and a clear statement of their mission.

External links

- Continua Health Alliance website [1]
- American Telemedicine Association [13]
- MobiHealthNews [14]
- Telemedicine History [15]
- Association of Telehealth Service Providers [16]

See also

- Connected Health
- eHealth
- Telehealth
- Telemedicine
- Health 2.0

References

[1] http://www.continuaalliance.org
[2] http://www.continuaalliance.org/about-the-alliance.html
[3] http://www.continuaalliance.org/static/cms_workspace/Continua_Version_One_Design_Guidelines_Now_Available_final.pdf
[4] http://continuaalliance.org/news-and-media/press-releases/founding-continua.html
[5] http://continuaalliance.org/static/binary/cms_workspace/Continua_Update_release_v_FINAL_2_.pdf
[6] http://continuaalliance.org/certified-products/nonin-2500-palmsat%C2%AE-pulse-oximeter.html
[7] http://www.nonin.com/News.aspx?NewsID=86
[8] http://www.continuaalliance.org/products/certified-products.html
[9] http://www.continuaalliance.org/static/cms_workspace/Continua_06082009_vFINAL.pdf
[10] Member Companies (English) (http://www.continuaalliance.org/about-the-alliance/member-companies.html)
[11] Board of Directors (English) (http://www.continuaalliance.org/about-the-alliance/board-of-directors.html)
[12] http://continuaalliance.org/static/cms_workspace/Continua_Overview_Presentation_v15_3.pdf
[13] http://www.americantelemed.org/i4a/pages/index.cfm?pageid=1
[14] http://mobihealthnews.com/
[15] http://www.depts.ttu.edu/communications/vistas/archive/02-summer/stories/miracle-of-telemedicine.php
[16] http://atsp.org/default.asp

Article Sources and Contributors

Telecare *Source*: http://en.wikipedia.org/w/index.php?title=Telecare *Contributors*: -fin, Alinja, Argon233, AvicAWB, Calltech, CliftonRugby, Darrelljon, David111180, Geologyguy, Iridescent, Karstenandjason, Mild Bill Hiccup, OlEnglish, Paul foord, Pgillman, Presnser, Qingostarr, Rsabbatini, Sgkay, Speechpathology, Stillplaygbc, Technopat, TelecareTechnology, Tleckie, Uncle Dick, 23 anonymous edits

Sensor *Source*: http://en.wikipedia.org/w/index.php?title=Sensor *Contributors*: 01101001, 12st12st12, 16@r, A.K., AK Auto, Achalmeena, Alexandrov, Allstarecho, Alteripse, Amaltheus, AmyKondo, Analogauthority, Andrewpmk, Anlace, Anthony Appleyard, AntonioSajonia, Ashoksharmaz87, Atlan, Atlantia, Atul44885, Axel.mulder, Barkeep, Beetstra, Benvogel, BillC, Binksternet, Blainster, Blobglob, Bobo192, Boing! said Zebedee, Bongwarrior, CENSI, Calltech, Caltas, Caltrop, Can't sleep, clown will eat me, CanadianLinuxUser, Capricorn42, Chaosdruid, ChemGardener, Clan-destine, Cowman109, Cpl Syx, D climacus, DH85868993, DanaRuff, Dancter, Darth Panda, Dawnseeker2000, Dbcv, Decltype, DerHexer, Dhiva1, Diannaa, Dicklyon, Dieselbub, Digresser, Dina, Dmr2, E Wing, ERK, Eaolson, Edebraal, Ehynes, Electricsforlife, EncMstr, Epbr123, Eric119, Evilrabidplotbunnies, EyeSerene, Fabartus, Falcon8765, Femto, Finejon, Flowerpotman, Funandtrvl, Galoubet, Geekstuff, Gene93k, Geodesic42, Giftlite, Gilliam, Glaurung, Glenn, GoingBatty, GrayFullbuster, Green-eyed girl, Grubber, Guidod, Gzkn, HalfShadow, Hankwang, Harriv, Haukurth, Helix84, Henkjanvanderpol, Heron, Hukseflux, Iamjp180, Iautomation, Ikalogic, Indurilo, Jackelfive, Jaeger5432, Jaxhere, Jc3s5h, Jlmerrill, Jni, JoanneB, Jon Awbrey, JonHarder, Jondel, Jreferee, Karafias, Kaverin, Keyence, Kingpin13, Kisss256, Kkolodziej, KnowledgeOfSelf, Korg, LOL, LeaveSleaves, Leonard G., Levineps, Light current, Lights, Love Krittaya, Mac, Madurasn, Mako098765, Malo, Manavbhardwaj, Mark Kretschmar, Masgatotkaca, MauriceKA, Mdd, Meaghan, Meekywiki, Mesdale, Metricopolus, Mikr18, Minakshimeena, Mion, Miroslavpohanka, Momergil, Momo san, Monkey230, Mortenoesterlundjoergensen, MrOllie, Mrh30, NawlinWiki, Ncmvocalist, Neelix, Nemilar, Newbi, Nick Alexeev, Nornen3, Nposs, Oli Filth, Omair.majid, Onebravemonkey, Ot, Patrick, Patrick Berry, Pavithrabtech, Payno, Pb30, Pearle, Peruvianllama, Petrb, Phantom784, Phemanth88, Pigletpoglet, Pit, Pro66, Publunch, Qatter, R'n'B, RJFJR, Raasgat, Rabbiz, Radudobra, RainbowOfLight, Rajeev1988, RalphWiggum, Rdsmith4, Renaissancee, Rettetast, ReturnofPenitron, Rigadoun, Rpyle731, Rubin joseph 10, Sadik ulubey, Sanders muc, Sapphic, Semiwiki, Sergio.ballestrero, Shadowjams, Shawnhath, SilentC, Silivrenion, Sinbaddasail0r, Sir Nicholas de Mimsy-Porpington, Sjorford, Slowking Man, Smack, Snowdog, Snowolf, Solarmicrowavefive, Sole Soul, Sonett72, Sourcer66, Squidonius, Srleffler, Stephenb, Steve Pucci, Stoneygirl45, Stuartfost, SuperMono, Sven Manguard, Synthy, The Anome, The Photon, The flamingo, TheFeds, Thubing, Tiddly Tom, TigerShark, Tohd8BohaithuGh1, Tommy2010, Troy.peterson, Ummairsaeed, V8rik, Vactivity, Vanished User 8a9b4725f8376, Veinor, Vsmith, West.andrew.g, WikHead, WikiLeon, Wikifan798, YourEyesOnly, Z4ngetsu, ZX81, Zzuuzz, 468 anonymous edits

Dementia *Source*: http://en.wikipedia.org/w/index.php?title=Dementia *Contributors*: 16@r, 2005, 28421u2232nfenfcenc, 3210, ACEOREVIVED, AJsMom, Aaron Kauppi, Abd, Abid0409, Acdwiki, Acroterion, Adamsacres, Adrian 1001, Aenioc, Ageingresearch, Ajorm, AlCapwned707, Alansohn, Alex.muller, AlexOlsen, AlexiusHoratius, Alexrexpvt, Alicecwj, Allstarecho, Amaher, Amakuru, AndrewScheuber, Anthonyhcole, Aranel, Arcadian, Aronian, Aspire3623WXCi, Atulsnischal, Auricfuzz, Avenged Eightfold, AxelBoldt, AxiomShell, Badgettrg, Badman15, Bagworm, Bbucks, Beland, Bemoeial, Ben Slijkhuis, Benbest, Betacommand, Bewildebeast, Bhod, BillC, Blankcortex, Blobcat, Bob247, Bobo192, Bobrayner, Bogey97, Bongwarrior, Boo821, Brewhaha@edmc.net, Brick Thrower, Brjaga, Bubba73, Bunnyhop11, Burnte, Bussys, CNicol, Caesarjbsquitti, Calltech, Candiman45, CanisRufus, Capnjim123, Capricorn42, Casliber, Casurr1, Cat Cubed, Cbustapeck, Charity6ks, CheesemonkeyFrenchperson, Cheryl Nash, Chimesmonster, Chris Capoccia, Chris the speller, Chrisjameshull, Chrispounds, Chzz, Cindelle, Citruscyanide, Ckatz, CliffC, Closedmouth, CloudSurfer, Cntras, Coder Dan, CombatCraig, Confiteordeo, Contentmaven, Countincr, Cowcilll, Craigsjones, Crisis, CrookedAsterisk, Culturejam, Curehd, Cymsdale, Damwiki1, DanielCD, Davejohnsan, Daveswagon, David Justin, Davidjonsson, Davidruben, Ddickson33, DeadEyeArrow, Debresser, Deedubzed, Deli nk, DeltaQuad, DerHexer, Dgijdeyoung, Dhj davis, Diberri, Discospinster, Distal24, Doczilla, Dougofborg, Download, Dr.alf, Drahcir, Dreamyshade, Drgarden, Drphilharmonic, Dvmedis, Earlypsychosis, Edgar181, Egil, Eiler7, Eleassar, Enter the PHiL, EoGuy, Epastore, Epbr123, Ephilei, Eras-mus, Erebus555, Everything Else Is Taken, Expertcoder, Falcon8765, Feelsky, Fenice, FiachraByrne, FisherQueen, Forbunk, Fourthords, Frankie0607, GHe, Gadfium, Gakusha, Garrondo, Gaurav1146, Geb11, GenOrl, General Tojo, GhostInTheMachine, Gilliam, Gimmetrow, Globeliner, Gobonobo, Gogo Dodo, GraemeL, Grahammc81, Grandmagrouper, Grcampbell, GreatWhiteNortherner, GrooveDog, Guillaume2303, Gwernol, H Padleckas, Habj, Hadel.tabayoyong, Haham hanuka, HalfShadow, Hd1968, Headbomb, Hede2000, Hmains, Hooray Henry, Hordaland, Hraefen, Huggle, Hut 8.5, Ivan Bajlo, J.delanoy, JForget, Jamisonhalliwell, Jan eissfeldt, Jason Quinn, Jauhienij, Jaytekz, Jerry, Jeversol, Jfdwolff, Jfitzg, JimVC3, Jloomis007, Jmh649, Johan1298, JohnPaulPagano, JonHarder, Jonathan Hall, Jonkerz, Jorvik, JoshuaZ, Julesd, Julia68, JulieADriver, K.GPCOG, Kafziel, Kanags, Kevinpurcell, KnowledgeOfSelf, Konstable, Krash, L Kensington, Lambiam, Lamekid45, Larocka, LeadSongDog, Leafyplant, Leevanjackson, Les boys, Lightmouse, Lindsey.tremulis, Literaturegeek, Lord Emsworth, Lowellian, Ltnature, Lumanog.n, M.Nagano, MER-C, Macclane64, Macdonald-ross, Mahleriavictim, MarloEditor, MartinPoulter, Mattisse, Mav, Maxis ftw, Mdineenwob, Mdwyer, Medtherapy, Mentifisto, Mephistophelian, Michael Hardy, Michele123, Miguelfenton73, Mikael Häggström, Mike2vil, MikeHydro, Miniapolis, MitchMcM, Mmortal03, Moomoomoo, Morrad, Mr little irish, Msikma, Mstaude01, Mudassar Zia, Mushroom, Mylesclough, Mystyc, Natebarratt, Nbauman, Neilbeach, Neurotip, Neutrality, Nicky.gregory, Nifty nobu, Notedgrant, Notepadpage, Nutriveg, Nuujinn, Obrienbr, OccupationalTherapist, Odyseuss123456, Ohconfucius, Ojigiri, Opelio, Opmh, Orangemarlin, Oskar71, Osm agha, Owen, Pakaran, Panboom, Paradigm Shift, ParisianBlade, ParlorGames, Pathoschild, PeterTheWall, Peterhuang77, Philip Trueman, Plasticup, Pleasantville, Pope Tetsuo, Progressiveneuro, PsyDisorderly, PsychEDUInfo, Quest for Truth, R500Mom, RDBrown, RG2, RainbowOfLight, Rash, Raymond murphy, Rdelagram, Recognizance, Regre7, Rettetast, RexNL, Rhombus, Rich Farmbrough, Rich Janis, Rjwilmsi, Rockstar915, RoyalIMD, Rrburke, Rsobrien390, Rubbrchikin, Ryulong, SJP, SMC, Sallison, Sannse, Saumyamittal, Sbharris, SchfiftyThree, Scwlong, Sean Lute, Sean.hoyland, Sertrel, Shadowjams, Shaliron, Shandris, Sharkb, Shawisland, Shnishna, Shoessss, SilkTork, Sim, Siodaoconnor, Sirs decades, Sjakkalle, Skarebo, Slightsmile, Smartse, Smyth, Snowmanradio, Species2112, SpikeTorontoRCP, Sproutamc, Stephen Allison, Steve M26, Steven Zhang, Strake, Susan. muzondo, Syleth, TUF-KAT, Tarotcards, Techdoctor, The Thing That Should Not Be, TheNewMessiah, Thedementiacentre, Theherald1000, Thesis4Eva, Tide rolls, Timwi, Tlesher, Tonythiru, Tonywalton, Topbanana, Treisijs, TucsonDavid, Turlis04, Tzepish, Uberplauge23, Una Smith, Unschool, Vaughan, Veinor, Vphanko, Vranak, Wavelength, West Brom 4ever, Wfeidt, WhisperToMe, Wik, Wikiklrsc, Wikipedarat, Will Beback, William Avery, Willking1979, Wouterstomp, Wtmitchell, Xa!, Xil, Yamamoto Ichiro, Yerpo, Yintan, Yobol, Zidane tribal, Zigger, Ziphon, Кайдзен, דניאל55, 614 anonymous edits

Safety_Confirmation *Source*: http://en.wikipedia.org/w/index.php?title=Safety_Confirmation *Contributors*: Presnser, 9 anonymous edits

Telemedicine *Source*: http://en.wikipedia.org/w/index.php?title=Telemedicine *Contributors*: A. B., AbsolutDan, Aiko, Alib, Allenplanet, Anriz, Apparition11, Arcadian, Argon233, Audiosmurf, AustralianMelodrama, Az1568, Badgettrg, Balsamfir, Barek, Basmah79, Bjerrk, Broadband118, Carl.bunderson, Carlitosau, Celtic fairies, Ceyockey, Chillin69x, Chris the speller, Closedmouth, Cobaltbluetony, DOC DS, Danapsimer, Davidcohen, DerHexer, Deville, Dgilperez, Diannaa, Dibnisha, Disasterlogistics, Drkhalifa, Dtolj, EBMdoc, EditingFrenzy, Eilily, Escape Orbit, Etayvas, GB fan, GRBerry, GRIFFEY366, Gauri Batra, GenOrl, Hadal, Harryzilber, Headbomb, HenryLi, Heron, Ianalis, Infrogmation, Interoperable, Iridescent, JHMM13, JivaGroup, Jleder, JonHarder, Jwcknet, KAErps, Karl.brown, Kate, Kauczuk, Kku, KnowledgeOfSelf, Kubanczyk, Kunalkhurana1, Lboehner-ejohnson, Lenapi, Lenapi2009, Light current, MAgrell, Mamurphy88, Martarius, Mco44, Mebrooks1969, Mereda, Middayexpress, Mini-Geek, Mochachocca, Mootros, Mpulier, MrOllie, Mrnicksmith, Mtavella, Mukherjiarnab, Nan KT, NatureBoyMD, Neon369, Ngtm, Nixeagle, Novangelis, Ohnoitsjamie, Omicronpersei8, Onco p53, Paddles, Paf25, Pak21, Paperclip777, Pch123, Phaedrus86, Piano non troppo, Piotrus, Pvosta, R'n'B, Rich Farmbrough, Riteview, Robert A West, Rsabbatini, Ryansean, SGogia, Sbbhattacharyya, Scatter22, Scjessey, Shanafme, Shltn, Slipstream, Slugmaster, Spotharaju, Spsood, Stanqo, Sterling.M.Archer, Stuartyeates, Sumsum2010, Sunidesus, Supten, Thenthorn, Thielst, Tiggerjay, Tmulak, Torbinsky, Velella, Vgprak, Wanscher, Wavelength, We hope, WikHead, Wmahan, WurmE, YSSYguy, Yazmínmx3, Zeeshanchattha, Zubinthakore, 249 anonymous edits

Telehealth *Source*: http://en.wikipedia.org/w/index.php?title=Telehealth *Contributors*: Ahmadr, Amy D. Schubert, ArmadilloFromHell, Barek, Blewisopensystemsmedia, Bmludwig, Bobo192, Books fan, BrownHairedGirl, Bslewis1, CDN99, Camerong, Canyonchaser, Cassiemarantz, Ceyockey, Chasingsol, DARTH SIDIOUS 2, Danny.j.wood, Df1002, Dirk Koekemoer, Dondegroovily, Dtolj, Edmondramly, Eilily, Erianae, Escape Orbit, Frankie, GRIFFEY366, Glengold, Gogo Dodo, HMMcat, Harryzilber, HenryLi, Interoperable, Iridescent, JDDC1, JKofoed, Jamesfreeman404, Jessica72, Jleder, John.coleman24, JohnDavidson, Journalist1983, Karl.brown, Khcf6971, Kheerand, Lavanian, LordAbernathy, Luchital, Margin1522, Markhurd, MattKingston, Mike Rosoft, Mpulier, MrOllie, Mrnicksmith, Nan KT, NatureBoyMD, Ngtm, Novangelis, Pak21, PaulWicks, Pearle, Phyton 2, PigFlu Oink, Piotrus, Pvosta, Rabinowitz, Redfarmer, Rich Farmbrough, Riggs77, Riteview, Robina Fox, Rougue scholar, Rsabbatini, Ryanphonetophone, SDaley2010, Sethdillon, Shltn, Shyamdash, Slon02, Slp1, SpuriousQ, THB, TNHNS, Tbulger, Telehealth, Theroadislong, Tma-medical, Versageek, Wavelength, Woohookitty, Xenva, Your Lord and Master, ZayZayEM, 116 anonymous edits

ECare_(software) *Source*: http://en.wikipedia.org/w/index.php?title=ECare_%28software%29 *Contributors*: Bearcat, Dawynn, Kathleen.wright5, Malcolma, Msilverman, OlEnglish, Shinton, 1 anonymous edits

Assistive_technology *Source*: http://en.wikipedia.org/w/index.php?title=Assistive_technology *Contributors*: 2over0, AVRS, Abilitynet, Abortman, Acecliffy, Aceituno, Acroterion, Alan Pascoe, Alasdairking, Anbaolach, Andy Fugard, Angryapathy, Argon233, Atif.t2, Axistive, BD2412, Baiwy, Benjamin Hawkes-Lewis, Berthelemy, Bgcaus, Bluephoenixmedia, Brashear, Bryan Derksen, Calltech, Caltrop, Cander0000, Card54, Cdsjeff, Charlie Danger, Chocolateboy, ChristopheS, Cjs5177, Conversion script, Coroberti, Crazytales, DKqwerty, Damian Yerrick, Danielspencer91, Darrelljon, David Shay, DennisHC, Dennishc, Derek Ross, DougsTech, Drbreznjev, Edward, Eileenspringer, Epbr123, Failedwizard, Fama Clamosa, Fastily, Femto, Ferox Seneca, Flatterworld, Frecklefoot, Free Bear, Gaius Cornelius, Gmoscoso, Gorodnichy, GraemeL, Hersfold, Hunting dog, Ida Shaw, JJblack, JLaTondre, Ja 62, Jacksmack76, James Kemp, James-davis, Janezp, Jannaz, Jbtrout, Jeremydesouza, Jimfbleak, Jmabel, Jmarchn, Joeman, Jonathanawhite, Kat384, Kgeza7, Kgroth, Kikodawgzzz, Kmontgo, Kurykh, Kyorosuke, Larry Hardesty, Larry_Sanger, LeadSongDog, Lindsey10, Lintzee1034, Lochneil, MZMcBride, MarkThomas, Martarius, Mcrasmusson, Mdrejhon, Merelake, Miniapolis, Mirokado, MrVibrating, Natgoo, Nemo19, Nfsjunkie91, NorthernThunder, NotACow, One Salient Oversight, Orphan Wiki, OverlordQ, Panfakes, Patricktimony, PaulLargo, Paulmcdonald, Peruvianllama, Pgillman, Pmd1991, PsychTalker, Qingostarr, RDBrown, RadekC, Reason turns rancid, Rich Farmbrough, Rjwilmsi, Rltodd, Robert of Ramsor, Robsavoie, RodC, Ronz, Rwdsp09, Saccades, Sam Hocevar, Sc2020, Schogla, Shadowjams, Shatner2011, Sigma 7, Sitara9, Slon02, Srleffler, StAnselm, Surabian, Suruena, Technopat, TelecareTechnology, TheRollingRock, Tide rolls, Tregoweth, Ukot, VegitaU, Vquex, Vsmith, Wavelength, Wibbz, Wighson, Wikilwalk, Willwade, Wmahan, 244 anonymous edits

Wandering_(dementia) *Source*: http://en.wikipedia.org/w/index.php?title=Wandering_%28dementia%29 *Contributors*: AlzWebTeam, Ammowriter, Betswiki, Ckatz, Coder Dan, GVnayR, Gregbard, Killiondude, Matt Lewis, Medtherapy, Ms26416, My secure locker, Notedgrant, Pigman, Qingostarr, State of Love and Trust, Tabletop, Una Smith, Whatever404, 15 anonymous edits

Remote_therapy *Source*: http://en.wikipedia.org/w/index.php?title=Remote_therapy *Contributors*: Haruth, Luchital, Rich Farmbrough, WhatamIdoing

Biotronik *Source*: http://en.wikipedia.org/w/index.php?title=Biotronik *Contributors*: Alawa, Ceyockey, Cntras, Medtechmonitor, Peter Karlsen, Trident13, 6 anonymous edits

Telemental_Health *Source*: http://en.wikipedia.org/w/index.php?title=Telemental_Health *Contributors*: Aaron Kauppi, Amalas, FiachraByrne, Rougue scholar, Rsabbatini, Rvitelli, Tbulger, Whitejay251, 2 anonymous edits

Telenursing *Source*: http://en.wikipedia.org/w/index.php?title=Telenursing *Contributors*: Alejotheo, Amy D. Schubert, Bunnyhop11, Earlypsychosis, Harryzilber, Jsfouche, Kiwi128, RJFJR, Rsabbatini, Steve carlson, THB, TenPoundHammer, The Rambling Man, 11 anonymous edits

Telepathology *Source*: http://en.wikipedia.org/w/index.php?title=Telepathology *Contributors*: Arthur Holland, Boing! said Zebedee, Carturo222, Deltaseeker, Harryzilber, KAErps, OlYeller21, Pascal666, R'n'B, RSWeinstein, Rdowney14, Rjwilmsi, TransporterMan, 15 anonymous edits

Telephone_triage *Source*: http://en.wikipedia.org/w/index.php?title=Telephone_triage *Contributors*: (aeropagitica), Alvestrand, Amy D. Schubert, Clicketyclack, Erechtheus, Jsfouche, Pearle, Printerbuilder, RJFJR, Rsabbatini, Scottalter, Steve carlson, Teletriage, 5 anonymous edits

Telepsychiatry *Source*: http://en.wikipedia.org/w/index.php?title=Telepsychiatry *Contributors*: Afishkind, Alansohn, Anna Lincoln, Bddmagic, Belovedfreak, Chris Capoccia, Gobonobo, Homepsychiatry, Philip Trueman, Rougue scholar, Rsabbatini, Supten, Welsh, 6 anonymous edits

Teleradiology *Source*: http://en.wikipedia.org/w/index.php?title=Teleradiology *Contributors*: Aesopos, AidenRyan, Alansohn, Apparition11, Arcadian, Asharafshahi, AvicAWB, Blabberhand, Ciscoperin, Davecrosby uk, Dekisugi, FauxClaud, FreplySpang, Greasybackflop, Hercule, Hibana, Ithilias, Jeepersjoseph, Jkeirn, Jmoock, Kukini, Lamro, McSly, Michaelmdx, Mitesh harlalka, MrOllie, Mwarf, Ourhistory153, Paf25, Radiologygenius, Rickwjenn, Riteview, Ronz, Rsabbatini, Shanetapper, Sueotis, Usteleradiology, WAvegetarian, WhatamIdoing, WikHead, Woohookitty, Wouterstomp, Wyatt915, 127 anonymous edits

Telerehabilitation *Source*: http://en.wikipedia.org/w/index.php?title=Telerehabilitation *Contributors*: Acebrock, B Pete, Barkeep, Briancua, Colinlee, Dbrienza, Ecohn, Fæ, Hargle, Harryzilber, J04n, Janezp, Jeff3000, Jlittlet, Jn.mdel, Joel7687, Josh Parris, Koavf, Mysoberlife, Obracy, Oli Filth, PGPirate, Piotrus, Rich Farmbrough, Rsabbatini, RyanGerbil10, STHayden, Sam Blacketer, Skysmith, Suepalsbo, SummerPhD, Sunidesus, Uanfala, Woohookitty, Zvar, 19 anonymous edits

The_Continua_Health_Alliance *Source*: http://en.wikipedia.org/w/index.php?title=The_Continua_Health_Alliance *Contributors*: Acutetech, AppForCalPERSMCII, BuffaloConspiracy, Castlewalk, Chowbok, Chris the speller, Continua, Ferritecore, Flowanda, FlyHigh, G825e3, Interoperable, JHunterJ, Jim.henderson, Kirkewing, Maelwys, Malcolma, MrOllie, Rsabbatini, Rwwww, The Rambling Man, Vegaswikian, VirtualizationGuru, Wayne Miller, WikHead, Wireless friend, Wtshymanski, 7 anonymous edits

Image Sources, Licenses and Contributors

File:Type K and type S.jpg *Source*: http://en.wikipedia.org/w/index.php?title=File:Type_K_and_type_S.jpg *License*: unknown *Contributors*: Skatebiker, 3 anonymous edits

Image:Alzheimer and other dementias world map - DALY - WHO2002.svg *Source*: http://en.wikipedia.org/w/index.php?title=File:Alzheimer_and_other_dementias_world_map_-_DALY_-_WHO2002.svg *License*: unknown *Contributors*: User:Lokal_Profil

File:US Navy 060518-N-2832L-013 Senior training specialist with Multi-Services Group International (MSGI), Michael Bedwell, trains Sailors to use Battlefield Medical Information Systems Telemedicine (BMIST) equipped Personal Digital.jpg *Source*: http://en.wikipedia.org/w/index.php?title=File:US_Navy_060518-N-2832L-013_Senior_training_specialist_with_Multi-Services_Group_International_(MSGI),_Michael_Bedwell,_trains_Sailors_to_use_Battle *License*: unknown *Contributors*:

Image:CT viewer Chest Keosys.JPG *Source*: http://en.wikipedia.org/w/index.php?title=File:CT_viewer_Chest_Keosys.JPG *License*: unknown *Contributors*: User:Mco44

File:Hoergeraet analog 050609.jpg *Source*: http://en.wikipedia.org/w/index.php?title=File:Hoergeraet_analog_050609.jpg *License*: unknown *Contributors*: User:Nordelch

Image:Accessible Cross.JPG *Source*: http://en.wikipedia.org/w/index.php?title=File:Accessible_Cross.JPG *License*: unknown *Contributors*: Eddau, Hebrew Wikipedia

Image:Head-wand.jpg *Source*: http://en.wikipedia.org/w/index.php?title=File:Head-wand.jpg *License*: unknown *Contributors*: User:Joebeone

Image:Sip-and-puff device.jpg *Source*: http://en.wikipedia.org/w/index.php?title=File:Sip-and-puff_device.jpg *License*: unknown *Contributors*: User:Joebeone

File:AAC user using eye gaze.JPG *Source*: http://en.wikipedia.org/w/index.php?title=File:AAC_user_using_eye_gaze.JPG *License*: unknown *Contributors*: Poule (talk). Original uploader was Poule at en.wikipedia

File:Continua registered logo.JPG *Source*: http://en.wikipedia.org/w/index.php?title=File:Continua_registered_logo.JPG *License*: unknown *Contributors*: Continua

MIX
Papier aus verantwortungsvollen Quellen
Paper from responsible sources
FSC® C105338

Printed by Books on Demand GmbH, Norderstedt / Germany